D1124668

Nursing Rural America

• • • • •

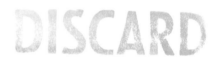

John C. Kirchgessner, PhD, RN, PNP, is a nurse historian whose research has focused on the nursing profession during the first half of the 20th century. His research explores the relationship between nurses and industry, specifically the work of nurses and the care they provided to West Virginian coal miners and their families. He has written and presented extensively on the West Virginia miners' hospitals, the 1907 Monongah Mine disaster, and public health in coal mining towns during the 1930s and 1940s. In addition, Dr. Kirchgessner has investigated how hospitals' nursing departments during the mid-20th century were often income generators for their respective institutions, not the cost centers administrators typically had claimed. He is an assistant professor of nursing at St. John Fisher College, Rochester, New York, and assistant director of the Eleanor Crowder Bjoring Center for Nursing Historical Inquiry at the University of Virginia, Charlottesville, Virginia. Dr. Kirchgessner co-authored *The Voice of Professional Nursing Education: A 40-Year History of the American Association of Colleges of Nursing,* has written book chapters, has published in refereed journals, and his research has been presented at international and national research meetings. Dr. Kirchgessner is a member of Sigma Theta Tau and the American Association for the History of Medicine, and is the newly elected second vice president of the American Association for the History of Nursing.

Arlene W. Keeling, PhD, RN, FAAN, is the centennial distinguished professor of nursing at the University of Virginia (UVA) in Charlottesville, Virginia. She received three degrees from UVA (BSN, 1974; MSN, 1986; and PhD from the Graduate School of Arts and Sciences in 1992), all after completing her Diploma in Nursing at Mountainside Hospital School of Nursing (Montclair, New Jersey) in 1969. She is currently chair of the Department of Acute and Specialty Care, University of Virginia School of Nursing, Charlottesville, Virginia.

Dr. Keeling is also the director of the Eleanor Crowder Bjoring Center for Nursing Historical Inquiry at UVA, one of only a few major nursing history centers in the world dedicated to the preservation, research, and dissemination of the history of the nursing profession. She has served as president of the American Association for the History of Nursing, and is currently serving as co-chair of the Expert Panel on Nursing History of the American Academy of Nursing. She is known nationally and internationally for her work in nursing history.

Dr. Keeling is the author/co-author of award-winning books, including *Nursing and the Privilege of Prescription, 1893–2000* (2007); *Nurses on the Front Line: When Disaster Strikes, 1878–2010* (Springer Publishing Company, 2010); and *Rooted in the Mountains, Reaching to the World: Stories of Nursing and Midwifery at Kentucky's Frontier School, 1939–1989* (2012). Written with Anne Cockerham, this book was the winner of the *American Journal of Nursing* Book of the Year award for Public Interest and Creative Works, 2012.

Dr. Keeling teaches historical research methods and nursing history in the PhD program at UVA. The recipient of numerous grants and author of many articles, Dr. Keeling is interested in documenting nursing history to shape health policy today.

Nursing Rural America
Perspectives From the Early 20th Century

• • • • •

John C. Kirchgessner, PhD, RN, PNP
Arlene W. Keeling, PhD, RN, FAAN

Editors

SPRINGER PUBLISHING COMPANY
NEW YORK

362.104257
N974

Springer Publishing Company, LLC
11 West 42nd Street
New York, NY 10036
www.springerpub.com

Acquisitions Editor: Joseph Morita
Composition: S4Carlisle Publishing Services

The cover features a photograph of a public health nurse, circa 1927. Courtesy of the American Red Cross. All rights reserved in all countries.

ISBN: 978-0-8261-9614-9
e-book ISBN: 978-0-8261-9615-6

14 15 16 / 5 4 3 2 1

The author and the publisher of this Work have made every effort to use sources believed to be reliable to provide information that is accurate and compatible with the standards generally accepted at the time of publication. The author and publisher shall not be liable for any special, consequential, or exemplary damages resulting, in whole or in part, from the readers' use of, or reliance on, the information contained in this book. The publisher has no responsibility for the persistence or accuracy of URLs for external or third-party Internet websites referred to in this publication and does not guarantee that any content on such websites is, or will remain, accurate or appropriate.

Library of Congress Cataloging-in-Publication Data
Nursing rural America : perspectives from the early 20th century / John C. Kirchgessner, Arlene W. Keeling, editors.
    p. ; cm.
Includes bibliographical references and index.
ISBN 978-0-8261-9614-9—ISBN 0-8261-9614-4—ISBN 978-0-8261-9615-6 (e-book)
I. Kirchgessner, John C., editor. II. Keeling, Arlene Wynbeek, 1948- editor.
[DNLM: 1. Rural Nursing—history—United States. 2. History, 20th Century—United States. WY 11 AA1]
    RA771.5
    362.1'04257—dc23   2014010255

Printed in the United States of America by Gasch Printing.

9/16

Contents

Contributors

* * * * *

Rima D. Apple, PhD
Professor Emerita
University of Wisconsin–Madison
Madison, Wisconsin

Anne Z. Cockerham, PhD, CNM,
  WHNP-BC
Associate Dean for Midwifery
  and Women's Health
Frontier Nursing University
Hyden, Kentucky

Sarah White Craig, PhD(c), CCNS,
  CCRN, CSC
Doctoral Candidate
University of Virginia School
  of Nursing
Charlottesville, Virginia

Mary E. Gibson, PhD, RN
Associate Professor, General Faculty
University of Virginia School
  of Nursing
Charlottesville, Virginia

Arlene W. Keeling, PhD, RN,
  FAAN
The Centennial Distinguished
  Professor of Nursing
Director, Eleanor Crowder
  Bjoring Center for Nursing
  Historical Inquiry

University of Virginia School
  of Nursing
Charlottesville, Virginia

John C. Kirchgessner, PhD, RN,
  PNP
Assistant Professor
Wegmans School of Nursing
St. John Fisher College
Rochester, New York

Sandra B. Lewenson, EdD, RN,
  FAAN
Professor, Lienhard School
  of Nursing
Pace University
Pleasantville, New York

Melissa McIntire Sherrod, PhD,
  RN, NE-BC
Associate Professor
Harris College of Nursing
  and Health Sciences
Texas Christian University
Fort Worth, Texas

Foreword

IT IS INDEED AN HONOR AND privilege to welcome you to this important book documenting the nurses who practiced in rural America in the first 50 years of the 20th century. These were years of great change and stress for the citizens of the United States who were faced with pervasive industrialization, two world wars, the Great Depression, and a large migration to urban areas. The editors, Dr. John C. Kirchgessner and Dr. Arlene W. Keeling, present stories and illustrations that exemplify the work of rural nurses in various regions of the United States, showing how, with limited access and resources, these nurses met the health care challenges brought on by poverty, isolation, and distance. Each chapter depicts nurses facing and overcoming a multitude of challenges as they addressed the medical needs of rural Americans. With a sense of commitment to their patients and communities, these nurses identified overarching community health problems and used their skills and available resources to improve the health of their communities. It is within these stories that the true measure of American nursing can be seen. Clearly, the nurses practiced to the full extent of their licenses. The nurses' stories entice the reader to travel along with them as they overcame obstacles, solved problems, and used their ingenuity and fortitude for the sake of others.

This historical volume exemplifies and supports the theoretical concepts particular to rural people and rural nursing as it explains the paradoxical complexity of rural life. The rural nurses understood the local culture and did not want to change it but, rather, to enhance its strengths. Because of their spirit of acceptance and community cooperation, their outcomes were remarkable: fully immunized communities, a decrease in mortality rates, statewide health policy implementation, and growth in community pride. The resilience of these nurses and their communities serves as a source of professional pride for problems solved and health enhanced.

Mary S. Collins, PhD, RN, FAAN
Glover-Crask Professor of Nursing
Director, DNP Program
Wegmans School of Nursing
St. John Fisher College
Rochester, New York

Preface

ACCESS TO HEALTH CARE FOR people living in rural areas of the United States is a major societal concern today. In fact, more than 60 million U.S. citizens who reside in rural areas are in need of safe, affordable, and quality health care, and nearly one in five of those is uninsured.[1] With the passage of the Patient Protection and Affordable Care Act (ACA) in 2010, opportunities to address this societal problem became a reality. As of October 2013, rural citizens, like all other U.S. citizens, have the opportunity to purchase affordable health insurance through the health insurance marketplace. Because rural residents are often poor, they are more likely to be eligible for affordable insurance under the coverage expansion in those states expanding Medicaid.[2]

The ACA may take years to implement fully and cannot, of course, solve some of the issues of access to care in rural areas, such as extreme weather conditions, bad roads, and long distances between patient homes and health care centers. However, the ACA has served to raise public awareness of disparities in access to quality health care. It has also led to a resurgence of interest in recruiting physicians and nurses to work in rural areas.

The problem of health disparities among rural Americans is not new. Since the origin of the United States in the late 18th century, residents of rural areas have not had the same opportunities as those in urban areas to access physicians, nurses, hospitals and, particularly, specialty care. Examining the history of health care services in rural America can provide us with insight into how physicians and nurses provided care to rural citizens in the past. That insight can shape health policy today.[3]

Most Americans are familiar with the iconic image of the rural country doctor making house calls by horse and buggy in the late 19th century and in the early decades of the 20th century, making those rounds in a Model T Ford. Fewer people are aware of *nurses'* work in addressing the health care needs of men, women, and children in rural America in the first half of the 20th century, yet nurses played a major role in direct care delivery as well as in the areas of health promotion and disease prevention. Like physicians, nurses rode horses, took buggies, or rode in Model T Fords—and later Jeeps—to reach patients and their families living in remote, isolated rural areas. This book presents nine case studies of nurses' work in select rural areas of the United States between the years 1900 and 1950 to identify, describe, and analyze the role of nurses in providing care. It also examines the effects of gender, class, race, policy, time, and place on rural health care. The book describes how nurses practiced to the full extent of their educational preparation—more than half a century before the Institute of Medicine made that recommendation in its 2011 report *The Future of Nursing: Leading Change, Advancing Health*.[4] Using primary historical data as evidence, the authors explain how nurses in rural settings crossed geographic, economic, and cultural barriers to provide access to care, and how they served as advocates for their often disenfranchised patients. *Nursing Rural America: Perspectives From the Early 20th Century* is meant to be a companion book to nursing textbooks that provide philosophical and theoretical elements of rural nursing and rural health care. It provides supplementary reading through historical case studies, demonstrating how characteristics that define rural nursing today have their roots in history.

In Chapter 1, "Town and Country Nursing: Community Participation and Nurse Recruitment," Sandra B. Lewenson recounts the inception and development of the Red Cross Town and Country nursing service during the years 1912 to 1947, demonstrating how the American Red Cross undertook "an extensive and systematically organized service of nursing [to provide care] for scattered dwellers in rural regions."[5] Lewenson begins this chapter by describing the formation of a Red Cross rural service that nurse leader Lillian Wald proposed in 1908. The chapter goes on to describe the recruitment and education of nurses to staff the Town and Country Nursing Service, identifies the importance of community participation, and highlights the unique work of the rural public health nurse. Particular attention is paid to the problem of finding nurses to work in rural areas and the tensions that developed between the Town and Country Nursing Service and the national organization of the American Red Cross.

In this chapter Lewenson identifies difficult terrain, lack of transportation, the vast distances in rural areas, and the impact of severe weather as barriers to care. In addition, she describes the unique nature of rural public health nurses' work, illustrating how the nurses had to provide "whatever was needed." As Lewenson notes, rural nurses had to be accomplished in all aspects of public health; the public health nurse's work was framed by the needs of the community. Lewenson's historical findings support Jane Scharff's contemporary assertion about the nature and scope of rural nursing practice: "Rural nursing is *generalist* nursing, not to be mistaken for mundane, and includes an intensity of purpose that makes it distinctive."[6]

The situation in rural Wisconsin between 1915 and 1940 that Rima D. Apple examines in Chapter 2, "Public Nursing in Rural Wisconsin: Stretched Beyond Health Instruction," provides historical documentation of the fits and starts of early rural public health systems and how nurses managed to provide access to care within them. In rural Wisconsin, public health nurses visited patients who lived in small towns and isolated, widely scattered homesteads—"a long way from anywhere and pretty close to nowhere"[7]—in areas that lacked essential resources. There nurses encountered clients, especially European immigrants, who resisted any changes to their traditional, culture-bound practices. They also discovered other residents who were eager to embrace modern health care practices but lacked the financial resources to do so. Indeed, poverty was widespread. Sometimes faced with the possibility of losing their jobs because of local government budget cuts, and often faced with unexpected circumstances that challenged their ability to provide rural clients with what nurses considered appropriate health care, the nurses defended their worth and looked for innovative solutions. They negotiated great distances, financial constraints, and policy barriers, using common sense, good judgment, and ingenuity to bring critically needed health services and health education to a previously overlooked and underserved rural population.

In Chapter 3, "School Nursing in Virginia: Hookworm, Tooth Decay, and Tonsillectomies," Mary E. Gibson describes and analyzes the nurse's role in providing care to rural school children in the Commonwealth of Virginia during the first 30 years of the 20th century. The Instructive Visiting Nurse Association had first introduced school nursing in Richmond in 1909, later relinquishing school nursing to the city health department. By 1916, in an attempt to improve population health, Virginia's Bureau of Public Health Nursing focused its early efforts on school nursing as a way to reach the state's many diverse localities and the families within them.

In this chapter, Gibson's focus on the local nature of the public health response to the children's needs reveals the importance of *place* in the development of school nursing programs. Lack of sanitation, inadequate heating and lighting, and poor water quality were all hallmarks of rural Virginia schools, and reflected similar conditions in the children's homes. Moreover, obtaining funding for school nurses was a persistent problem. As Gibson notes, "School nursing continually relied on a combination of private and public funding," with philanthropic efforts underpinning much of the early Virginia State Health Department work. Despite these barriers, school nurses worked autonomously, relying on their own physical assessment skills to diagnose physical defects, minor illnesses, and dental problems in the children. They also implemented treatments for hookworm; assisted in tonsillectomy clinics; and taught rural families the basics of nutrition, sanitation, and child care. School nursing not only served to meet children's health needs, it also gave nurses an entrée into the families' lives.

Establishing trust with the local community was essential to rural nursing, and in Chapter 4, "Nursing in Schoolfield Mill Village: Cotton and Welfare," Sarah White Craig describes how the nurses accomplished that feat with poor Whites and Blacks in the southern cotton mill villages, using the Schoolfield company town as a case study. Expecting to do "industrial nursing" as it was practiced in the Northeast under the leadership of Lillian Wald, nurses employed by the cotton mills in small towns in the South more often addressed the public health needs of the community. There, practicing in a space between social work and nursing, but within the cultural and legal space of the Jim Crow South, they cared for mothers and babies; taught the basics of sanitation, nutrition, and disease prevention; and encouraged attention to safe practices in the mills.

Meeting the public health needs of West Virginia coal miners and their families in the 1930s was challenging to the state and to those who provided care. In Chapter 5, "Care in the Coal Fields: Promoting Health Through Sanitation and Nutrition," John C. Kirchgessner describes the public health system in the coal towns of West Virginia in the early 20th century as a "patchwork." Employer funds, state funds, and philanthropic generosity provided the financial resources for programs, while private practitioners and "company" physicians worked together to provide the necessary care.

During the King Coal Era, when coal became the sole source of fuel for the American railroad and shipping industries and the coal industry grew, health care for individual miners and their families improved. However, the public health infrastructure in many communities remained inadequate, as did the focus on public health problems. In contrast to mining disasters and catastrophic injuries, which were dramatic and well publicized, problems like poor sanitation, polluted water, inadequate housing, the prevalence of infectious diseases, and high infant and maternal mortality were far less visible. The State Department of Public Health addressed some of these. However, as was true in many other regions of the country, the health department was overburdened and understaffed. Much of the responsibility was left to the local government. In coal towns, the responsibility fell to the company doctors, the miners' hospitals, and the public health nurses.

Responding to these public health concerns, health officials, nurses, local physicians, and the coal industry itself initiated services to help decrease mortality and morbidity rates. Using the Koppers Coal Nursing Service as an exemplar, Kirchgessner shows how coal company owners fulfilled their social obligations by employing nurses in the mining communities.

Assisting physicians or working on their own, coal town nurses conducted health classes, screened school children, held prenatal clinics, responded to epidemics, and made periodic sanitation tours of the community. In this chapter, Kirchgessner demonstrates how the Koppers' nurses used their own ingenuity and practiced to the full extent of their knowledge, experience, and legal boundaries to overcome the barriers of geography, culture, and class in the rugged mountain locality.

In Chapter 6, "Mary Breckinridge and the Frontier Nursing Service: Saddlebags and Swinging Bridges," Anne Z. Cockerham examines the geographic, cultural, social, and professional challenges that frontier nurses faced between 1925 and the mid-1950s as they cared for patients in the remote eastern Kentucky mountains. There, maternal and infant morbidity and mortality rates were among the highest in the nation. In order to address these problems, Mary Breckinridge created the Frontier Nursing Service (FNS) in 1925, establishing the headquarters in Leslie County.

Working in a decentralized system of rural outpost clinics under Breckinridge's leadership, the FNS nurses provided direct care, preventive services, and midwifery expertise to the Appalachian residents. At first, riding on horseback to reach remote log cabins and, later, traveling in Jeeps, FNS nurses covered an area of approximately 700 square miles to care for nearly 10,000 people. Negotiating cultural differences in a community whose members valued self-reliance, stoicism, and home remedies, the nurses introduced 20th-century scientific medicine and nursing, coaxing mothers and fathers to vaccinate their children, allow tonsillectomies, or admit their family member to the hospital. Their aim, according to Mary Breckinridge, was to leave "no territory uncovered and no people uncared for."[8] The setting, the culture, and the dearth of physicians in this remote mountainous region challenged the FNS nurses to use the full extent of their knowledge and skill. They did so, often working alone and relying on standing physician orders, or collaborating with one of their nursing colleagues to provide the necessary care. Themes that emerge in this chapter are those of nurse autonomy, cultural sensitivity, and community participation.

Crossing the barriers of culture and poverty to provide care is especially important in migrant nursing, and in Chapter 7, "Migrant Nursing in the Great Depression: Floods, Flies, and the Farm Security Administration," Arlene W. Keeling describes and analyzes the nurse's role in caring for migrant farmworkers and their families in California during the Great Depression. In demonstration projects and, later in the 1930s in government-sponsored "suitcase camps," nurses played a central role as first-line providers, working with a great deal of autonomy as they practiced nursing to the full extent of their education and skill. The nurse's role was threefold: (1) to help the migrants keep healthy, (2) to keep migrants from spreading disease, and (3) to keep workers in the field. Through their actions and relationships with the migrants, the nurses raised the questions of whether access to health care was a right or a privilege, who was deserving of health care services, and who should make those decisions.

Access to care was particularly difficult in the oil fields of west Texas. In Chapter 8, "Nursing in West Texas: Trains, Tumbleweeds, and Rattlesnakes," Melissa McIntire Sherrod describes how one physician and his wife left their home in St. Louis in the late 1940s to set up practice in the oil boom town of Iraan, in the Trans-Pecos region of Texas, a remote 17,000-square-mile region of the state where oil field workers, ranch hands, and their families lived. Working conditions in the oil and the ranching industries were dangerous, and traumatic injuries were frequent. In this chapter Sherrod highlights some of the dramatic rescue efforts that the Sherrods undertook to provide care in an area where neither acute care nor emergency care services were readily available. She also describes the difficulties of finding reliable transportation and the problems of transporting critically ill patients over rough terrain.

The chapter also identifies the problem of the lack of formal public health programs in the Trans-Pecos region, going on to describe how the physician/ nurse couple was successful in improving infant care and immunization rates despite the lack of resources. Indeed, the Sherrods made a major contribution to the state's public health efforts, screening for tuberculosis, immunizing ranchers and farm families, and fighting against polio. Using their medical and nursing expertise, and engaging other members of the community, Judy and Alan Sherrod provided care to a diverse population in an isolated corner of west Texas. It was rural health care at its best.

Many of the problems of access to care that nurses faced in other areas of the country in the early 20th century are reviewed in Chapter 9, "Nursing the Navajo: Dust Storms and Gully Washouts." In this chapter, Arlene W. Keeling describes and analyzes nurses' work in the Four Corners region of the United States in the first half of the 20th century. There, field nurses working for the Bureau of Indian Affairs (later called the Indian Health Services) had to negotiate not only the extremes in weather, the great distances between patients, and the harsh environmental conditions, but also the Navajo culture. Working to the full extent of their education and expertise while simultaneously navigating dust storms, gully washouts, and cultural borderlands, Bureau of Indian Affairs nurses took charge and provided effective health teaching and disease treatment and prevention. Through their perseverance, the nurses worked effectively, overcoming countless barriers to bring medical and nursing services to this underserved rural population.

Themes that emerge in the nine case studies include many that are commonly identified in the rural public health literature today. Among these are the challenges of overcoming geographic barriers to care, cultural differences in rural communities, the lack of medical and nursing resources, fear and prejudice, and extremes in weather conditions. Autonomy in nursing practice, "generalist" nursing, self-reliance, a "can-do" attitude, role expansion, and the opportunity for diverse patient experiences emerge as additional themes, as does the importance of community participation and community acceptance.[9]

The book's significance is twofold. First, it documents the reality of rural nursing in several different areas of the country, as well as within populations of different ethnic origins in the first half of the 20th century, thereby filling a gap in health care history and hopefully bringing to life what is often described only in theoretical terms. Second, the book provides historical, primary source data that support concepts, theory, and practice in rural nursing today. No doubt, the stories from the past will resonate for those practicing in rural areas today. In some respects, not much has changed when one considers the importance of *place* in access to care. In other respects, a comparison of the importance of *time* between the 20th century and the 21st century illuminates a great deal of change: Telemedicine, Internet access, helicopter transport, and the creation of the critical access hospital have converged today to change the nature of access to care in rural areas.

A historical approach to rural nursing is unique, bringing complexity and context to the current discussion of the right to health care, the problems of access to care for rural citizens, and the budget debates that follow. By examining those issues through the lens of history, the book makes an important contribution to understanding rural nursing today—in fact, it shows the difference between "nursing in a sparsely populated rural setting" and integrated, creative, "rural nursing."[10] By engaging in this historical analysis and living first-hand the experiences of nurses in the early 20th century, readers can increase their depth of understanding of what it meant to be a rural nurse then, and what that might mean today.

NOTES

1. C. V. Sumaya, *Rural Populations and Health: Determinants, Disparities, and Solutions.* R. A. Crosby, M. L. Wendel, R. C. Vanderpool, & B. R. Casey (eds.) (San Francisco, CA: Jossey-Bass, 2012), 1–3. See also accessed May 12, 2013, http://www.hhs.gov/healthcare/facts/factsheets/2013/09/rural09202013.html

2. Sumaya, *Rural Populations and Health,* Accessed May 12, 2013, http://www.hhs.gov/healthcare/facts/factsheets/2013/09/rural09202013.html

3. Arlene Keeling and Mary Ramos, "The Role of Nursing History in Preparing Nursing for the Future," *Nursing and Health Care: Perspectives on Community* 16, 1 (January/February 1995): 30–34.

4. Institute of Medicine of the National Academies, *The Future of Nursing: Leading Change, Advancing Health* (Washington, DC: The National Academies Press, 2011).

5. Lillian Wald to Jacob Schiff in 1910, cited in Lavinia L. Dock, Sarah Elizabeth Pickett, Fannie F. Clement, Elizabeth G. Fox and Anna R. Van Meter, *History of American Red Cross Nursing* (New York, NY: Macmillan, 1922), 1213.

6. Jane E. Scharff, Chapter 16, "The Distinctive Nature and Scope of Rural Nursing Practice: Philosophical Bases," Charlene Winters (ed.), *Rural Nursing: Concepts, Theory and Practice*, 4th ed. (New York, NY: Springer Publishing Company, 2013), 241–258 (quote, 255).

7. Scharff, "The Distinctive Nature and Scope of Rural Nursing Practice," 2013, 243.

8. Mary Breckinridge, *Wide Neighborhoods* (Lexington, KY: University Press of Kentucky, 1952), 228.

9. Charlene Winters, *Rural Nursing* (2013).

10. Scharff, "The Distinctive Nature and Scope of Rural Nursing Practice," 2013, 257.

1
•••••

Town and Country Nursing: Community Participation and Nurse Recruitment

•••••

SANDRA B. LEWENSON

It seems to me particularly appropriate for the Red Cross society to undertake ultimately in America, an extensive and systematically organized service of nursing for the scattered dwellers in rural regions, such as we now find well developed in Great Britain and in Canada.[1]

AMERICAN RED CROSS RURAL NURSING SERVICE (1912 TO 1913)

IN 1908 LILLIAN WALD, DIRECTOR of the Henry Street Settlement in New York City, envisioned a well-organized structure within the American Red Cross (ARC) to support care in rural areas. In her mind, ARC's primary purpose had been to provide care during times of war and emergencies. These two goals, Wald reflected, were sporadic and gave the organization little to do in peace time.[2] To her way of thinking, the ARC could provide a much-needed and sustained service to communities around the country during times of war *and* times of peace. That year, Wald presented her suggestion at a meeting in New York City at the home of Mayor George McClennan. The purpose of that meeting was to promote camps for children with tuberculosis as part of a larger, international antituberculosis campaign initiated by the Red Cross. Wald believed her ideas about providing rural public health fit well within the goals of this campaign.[3]

A few more years passed before Wald's suggestion achieved success. That success was dependent in part on support from Jacob H. Schiff, a family friend of Wald's as well as a member of ARC's Board. In her 1910 letter, delivered by Schiff at the annual Red Cross meeting in Washington, DC, Wald outlined a plan for the ARC to organize a rural nursing service that would be "national in scope."[4] Wald's plan included the establishment of a Rural Nursing Service headquarters in Washington, DC, the utilization of trained nurses and traveling supervisors, and the development of local chapters led by community supervisors. In addition, her plan included recognition of the importance of financial support for the additional education that the nurses would need to be successful in rural settings.

Although Wald's appeal to the ARC was not immediately accepted, by December of 1911, when Jacob Schiff and Mrs. Whitelaw Reid, both philanthropic supporters of the ARC, provided funding for the establishment of a Red Cross rural nursing service, Wald's vision became a reality. The Committee on Rural Nursing was established. The Committee brought together several notable socially minded leaders interested in nursing and the ARC, including philanthropists Mabel Boardman (Chairman), Mrs. Whitelaw Reid, Mrs. William Draper, John M. Glenn, and Wickliffe Rose (educator and executive secretary of the Rockefeller Sanitary Commission); nursing leaders, Jane Delano (Vice-Chair), Lillian Wald, and Annie Goodrich; and Dr. Winford Smith and Surgeon J. W. Schereschewsky (from the Public Health Service). By February 1912, a subcommittee, made up of nurses Jane Delano, Annie Goodrich, Lillian Wald, and Fannie Clement, had developed the standards for practice and education for rural nurses. The ARC Rural Nursing Service was formally established on November 12, 1912, for a 1-year trial period. Public health nurse Fannie Clement served as its first superintendent.[5]

The First Year

The Committee on Rural Nursing met throughout the first year to determine other collaborative relationships. For example, it was decided that the ARC Rural Service would collaborate with the Metropolitan Life Insurance Company (MetLife). Under that arrangement, the ARC rural public health nurse who visited MetLife policy holders would be paid by both MetLife and the ARC.

The Committee also developed the qualifications they sought in nurses who applied to this new service. Acceptable candidates would: (a) have to meet the "requirements of the Red Cross for enrollment, except all reference to age"[6] and (b) show successful completion of a "course covering a four-month period, or one-half academic year, under the supervision of a recognized Visiting Nurse Association, and a recommendation of the Association."[7] Just as

Wald believed that education was crucial to both the health of the public as well as the development of the role of the public health nurse, the Committee agreed that rural public health nurses needed additional education. They also realized the difficulty they would face in attracting nurses to work in rural settings, especially nurses who had the experience necessary to provide the full range of services required.[8]

Keen on recruitment and retention of nursing staff, the Committee established a recommended salary between $60 and $100 per month and a 30-day annual vacation.[9] To advertise the positions available, they developed several circulars providing information about vacations, salaries, and educational requirements, and specifying that rural nurses were expected to have "knowledge of driving and riding horses and possibly the use of a bicycle."[10]

The recruitment of nurses, especially nurses willing to take the additional 4-month course in preparation for their work, was daunting. Mabel Boardman wrote to Wickliffe Rose, executive secretary of the Rockefeller Sanitary Commission, for advice, explaining how, "in spite of a large amount of work that Miss Clement has done, it is most difficult to secure applicants for the special 4-month course required. As Chairman of the Committee, I will be glad if you would suggest to me any further means of arousing

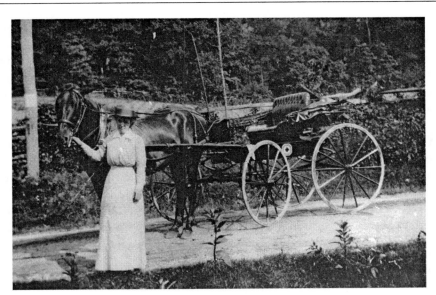

ARC public health nurse with horse and buggy in 1912.

● ● ● ● ●

interest among the nurses in this Rural Nursing Service."[11] Rose responded optimistically a few days later:

> With reference to the difficulty in interesting persons in making preparation for this rural nursing service I would suggest that you may find it very difficult to induce young women who have become accustomed to city life to accept service for the rural districts. It is my impression that you will find your best material in the country. In all our other work we find that people who have grown up in the country and who are now living in the country give us the best service in country work. When you can get the work started in a few centers you will have opportunity to bring the matter to the attention of young women who are now living in the country. The rural service itself will be your best means of securing recruits for the enlargement of the service. It is my impression that the real difficulty lies in getting the work started. That done, the rest will be increasingly easy.[12]

Community Participation

In order to implement the project at the local level, the Committee knew that community participation would be required. Mindful of the need to include community stakeholders in the introduction of rural public health nurses, the Committee carefully worded the ARC brochures to recommend that whenever the idea of starting a rural nursing service in a community arose, a "mass meeting of the whole community" be arranged so that these services could be explained and the needs of the community "emphasized."[13] The expense of starting such a venture would fall to the community, with the collection of membership fees or annual subscriptions to the nursing association.

An executive board for a local nursing association would be established in that community and it would be responsible for raising funds to support the nurses' salaries, to supply necessary items to be rented or loaned to patients when needed, and to arrange for hospitalization of patients when necessary. "No nurse, however valuable, will be able to accomplish good results in any community single-handed."[14] Cooperation and collaboration were expected of rural public health nurses, the community agencies, and the various stakeholders in the community's health.

Access to Care

Elizabeth Fox, director of the rural nursing service from 1921 to 1930, often described the challenges nurses faced while traveling miles over rugged and

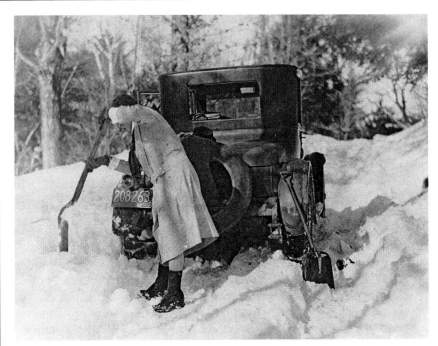

Public health nurse digging out car in snow in 1927.

● ● ● ● ●

isolated terrain to reach the families whom they served. Snow and sleet only complicated the situation.

ARC nurse, Christine Higgins, who was working in rural Maine at the Maine Missionary Society in 1921, wrote to her supervisor describing her experiences traveling from island to island with a team of other health professionals to provide health teaching and dental and medical care. According to that letter:

> . . . My uniform consists of rubber boots, army breeches, short skirt, flannel shirt and sheepskin-lined coat. The mud is very deep, boats have a faculty of being wet inside as well as outside, and the highways and byways of Cranberry Isle are not yet paved or even very wide or well marked in any way. Still we do have a Ford. I nearly collapsed when I heard it and expected a complete mental paralysis when I saw it. Really, expensive clothes are hardly the appropriate thing for this work. I clean house and build fires in the Community House every day. The

walking is at present very bad indeed, and the boat I came over in from North East Harbor was a combination fish and freight boat and I was glad of the warm but not expensive clothes which I had. . . . I am going to Islesford next week and then hope to have a horse for transportation. I shall be there two and possibly three weeks. . . . [15]

The Work

In addition to describing the hazards of travel, Higgins also wrote of the varied nature of rural public health nurses' work, noting: "Tomorrow I am to lead the Christian Endeavor Meeting, play the organ and give a little health talk. How's that!"[16] However, "all inclusive" as it was, the nurses' work was subject to regulations established by the ARC. Nurses were not expected to do night duty. Care for infectious patients was permitted only after ensuring that the nurse's other patients would be cared for by someone else. Attendance at normal births was permissible only if medical aid was unavailable. Records had to be completed using the report cards provided by the ARC. The nurse was to communicate directly with the physician in writing or in person rather than by leaving messages with patients. All nurses were supervised by the superintendent of rural nurses. Rural nurses served as the nursing reserve for the Army and Navy, helping during disasters and war. Finally, in addition to providing direct care, rural nurses were expected to "teach by instruction and demonstrations the principles of hygiene as applied to their homes and surroundings as well as of person."[17]

The work of the rural public health nurse was demanding. Those who opted for the rural setting found that their responsibilities required them to work within the community, travel great distances to visit their families, be teachers and facilitators of care, and offer whatever was needed in whatever way they could. At this local level nurses needed to be fluent in all aspects of public health. Fannie Clement, director of the newly formed ARC Town and Country Nursing Service, wrote frequently for the *American Journal of Nursing*, describing this innovative service and the work of the rural public health nurse:

I could give in detail, the report of a Red Cross Visiting nurse in a community of 1,000 population, largely foreign, among which last year she made 6,075 visits, besides doing 846 office dressings. Over half of the . . . visits were at the bedside and 400 of the balance were school nursing visits. This record . . . is exceptional. She has an automobile and every contrivance provided to make her work effective, yet what would this avail if back of it all, there did not lurk a most earnest purpose, a deep spirit of service as is that typified by our great National Red Cross in its endeavor through the medium of the visiting nurse, to alleviate suffering and promote genuine happiness in the homes of our rural people? . . .[18]

In the lumber camps established in New Hampshire along the Pemigawsett River, another ARC rural public health nurse provided classes in home hygiene and care of the sick for camp mothers. In addition, nurses traveled with physicians throughout the rural wilderness, engaging in "preventive work as well as actual nursing."[19] Conditions in the lumber camps— including unventilated housing, lack of immunizations, frost bite, and other complications related to communicable and other kinds of disease—directed the work of the nurse.[20]

The work of the public health nurse was framed by the needs of the community; the religious, ethnic, and racial makeup of that community; the kinds of preexisting public health care organizations; and the geographical location. Each Red Cross chapter, whether in the mountains of New Hampshire, or in Kentucky, or in the West, directed the kinds of work that the public health nurse would need to accommodate. The work ranged from bedside care for frost bite and the establishment of well-baby clinics, to school nursing, industrial nursing, the offering of classes in home hygiene and care of the sick, and providing educational and publicity about her work.[21]

Sometimes only one nurse was available in an area; at other times the nurse had additional public health nurses with whom to share the district. In either case, the nurse had to have skills in establishing close ties with the community in which she worked. Some towns preferred to place their own nurse rather than accept someone from outside their rural area. This preference often created tensions that needed to be resolved in order to ensure the success of the public health nursing service. Frequently it was the skill of the nurse that created the necessary compromise and resolution. The Red Cross tried to "fill the gaps in the health organization of the country and to blaze the trail in the unreached areas."[22] The success of these nurses relied on the ability of the ARC to recruit and retain public health nurses who were suitable for work in these rural settings. This concern remained a constant and enduring problem from the beginning of the ARC rural nursing service to its dissolution in 1947.

Additional Education for Rural Practice

Because of their varied responsibilities and the remoteness of the areas in which they worked, these dedicated rural public health nurses required additional education. Topics such as communication, sociopolitical and economic factors, cultural understanding, and social awareness were particularly important.[23] Thus, one of the major contributions of the Red Cross rural nursing service was the requirement of additional education. The existing hospital-based training programs did not prepare nurses to provide public health nursing services specific to urban settings or rural settings. It was in rural settings especially that nurses needed skills that only additional education could provide. The minimum ARC requirement of the additional 4-month course in public health nursing led to the establishment of new collegiate programs in rural health throughout the early 20th century.

Teachers College at Columbia University in New York City was considered the epitome of excellence in nursing education. Early on, the Committee on Red Cross Rural Nursing identified Teachers College as the exemplar for the new programs in rural health. In conjunction with Lillian Wald's Henry Street Settlement and the District Nursing Association of Northern Westchester, Teachers College developed a curriculum providing nurses with experiences in both rural and urban public health nursing. As early as 1914 and 1915, some of the postgraduate courses at Teachers College included practical sociology, municipal and rural sanitation, and public health nursing, which included a practicum in rural and urban public health.[24]

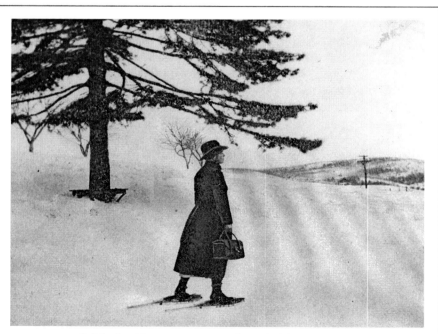

Public health nurse on snowshoes in Maine in 1920.

● ● ● ● ●

Insufficient Workforce

Finding nurses to work in rural areas was always a problem. Anticipating the difficulty the organization would have in attracting a sufficient number of public health nurses to work in isolated settings, Wald optimistically wrote:

> At first it would seem a most difficult matter to obtain suitable women for this work. I believe this is not insurmountable. The very existence of the association on so great a scale would stimulate the nurses in the training school. . . . It would probably develop that scholarships could be given to send specially fitted young women to the postgraduate course at Teachers College. . . . In my opinion, it would be much more desirable for the Red Cross society to take up this work than it would be to organize another national society, for reasons that are so obvious. I do not think the United States would need much stimulus, for I believe that the cause carries its own appeal.[25]

Aside from setting the standards for public health nurses, the Rural Nursing Service offered communities an affiliation that would provide them with qualified public health nurses who could support the existing community services, or assist communities in developing visiting nurse associations when needed. The ARC offered these communities "general supervision over its rural nurses," as well as provided some financial support for them.[26] The ARC expected the community affiliations to eventually be autonomous, but in order for an affiliation to occur, these communities and nurses had to meet the clearly stated "Conditions of Affiliation of Nursing Associations with the ARC" and "Regulations for Nurses."[27] Communities that wanted to deviate from the ARC's regulations, such as hire a nurse from within the community, would have to inform the ARC so that "a mutual understanding of the needs of a community" could be developed.[28] This relationship between the ARC and local communities proved too difficult at times, as the ARC wanted to maintain high standards and uniformity yet recognized that the communities had their own needs to consider. Just as tension arose on the issue of recruitment, this tension continued throughout the 36-year existence of the ARC's public health nursing programs.

By 1913, the ARC Rural Nursing Service culminated with a successful outcome, including "ten affiliated associations, appointment of a nurse for supervisory work in the Metropolitan Life Insurance Company, the establishment of Teachers College course for rural nurses . . . and an exhibit sent to Tulsa, Oklahoma."[29]

TOWN AND COUNTRY NURSING SERVICE (1913 TO 1918)

Following the successful first year of the ARC Rural Nursing Service, the name was changed to reflect an expansion of the public health nursing service to towns larger than just those in rural communities. In 1913 the experimental Rural Nursing Service became the Town and Country Nursing Service.[30] This new identity lasted until 1918 when again the name changed to reflect the growing needs of the American people following World War I (Table 1.1). Throughout the first 5 years of the Town and Country Nursing Service, the initial Committee expanded to include representation from three national nursing organizations, from the ARC, and from the laity. It continued to set the rules and regulations that directed the communities using the ARC rural public health nurse.[31]

At the 20th anniversary of the ARC's rural public health nursing service, Elizabeth Gordon Fox reflected on the growth of the service, writing: "One by one, to the southern mountains, to mining camps, to farming counties, to small towns, to an industrial village, went Red Cross nurses, often the first to undertake rural work in a given State, and with them went a constant stream of wise advice and encouragement."[32] Fox described the early years of the service as utopian, with three main goals that consisted of spreading the idea of the service around the country, recruiting qualified nurses as the demand for these professionals continued to rise, and providing sufficient support for "proper growth."[33] As the additional rural public health training was so vital to this organization, the ARC continued to seek opportunities for additional educational programs. At times their focus on education became a source of tension with competing organizations. The responsibility and control of nursing education became a divisive issue between the ARC and the newly formed National Organization for Public Health Nurses (NOPHN), founded

TABLE 1.1 American Red Cross Evolving Names

NAME	DATES	REASONS FOR CHANGE
Rural Nursing Service	1912–1913	1-year trial
Town and Country Nursing Service	1913–1918	Changed to Town and Country to include rural districts and smaller towns rather than just the rural districts
Bureau of Public Health Nursing	May 18, 1918–1932	Following the war they included cantonment zones where public health nurses were placed
Public Health Nursing and Home Hygiene and Care of the Sick	1932–1948	Combined the services of the public health nurse with ARC home hygiene and care of the sick program

in 1912. The leadership and membership of both groups overlapped, causing an ongoing debate over the goals and functions of both groups.

The minutes of the fourth meeting of the ARC's Committee on Rural Nursing suggested the possibility of the ARC uniting with the newly formed National Organization of Public Health Nursing (NOPHN) and the National League of Nursing Education (NLNE). Nurse leader Annie Goodrich suggested that a joint committee of these three organizations be established to address the issues related to training centers for public health nurses. The leaders of these organizations, Clara Noyes and Adelaide Nutting of the NLNE, and Mary Gardner and Elizabeth Crandall of the NOPHN, joined the committee and discussed the possibilities of "cooperation."[34] In that spirit of cooperation, the editors of the journal *Public Health Nurse* (the official organ of NOPHN), developed a section that provided public health nurses with information about the ARC's public health nursing service. In spite of that effort, tension between the two organizations emerged over time and grew significantly regarding the role they both would play in the rise of rural public health nursing.[35] In 1913 Lillian Wald addressed this increasing tension by writing to the Committee on Town and Country Nursing to define the scope of Town and Country and the NOPHN:

> . . . each has, in my judgment, a distinctive place and should interlock without overlapping, . . . the difference between the two societies, as I see it, is that the one is for education and mutual benefit, a union of workers and those interested in their work, and the other administrative and supervisory. In my judgment it would seem that our Red Cross Committee ought not to establish educational centers, but that it should send nurses who are to be enrolled in Red Cross work to the educational centers provided by other organizations. It ought to be the business of Teachers College and the National Organization for Public Health Nursing to promote these educational centers in the interest of public health nursing throughout the country.[36]

BUREAU OF PUBLIC HEALTH NURSING (1918 TO 1932) AND PUBLIC HEALTH NURSING AND HOME HYGIENE AND CARE OF THE SICK (1932 TO 1948)

With the start of World War I, qualified rural public health nurses became exceptionally scarce as the demands for nurses in the war exceeded the supply. But when the war finally ended, the service saw a "sudden and revolutionary change."[37] Many of the local chapters began focusing on community needs rather than only addressing the neediest community members. Communities not only found an increase in available Red Cross funds following the war, but they also saw an increase in the demand for rural public health nurses. Once again the title of the service changed. In 1918 the Town and Country Nursing Service became known as the Bureau of Public Health Nursing. The name reflected a broader role and responsibility as bureau nurses supported additional populations scattered in towns, rural settings, and even larger cities.[38] Public health nurse Mary Gardner replaced Fannie Clement as director, but her role was soon transferred to associate director Elizabeth G. Fox due to Gardner's work in Italy.[39] Fox remained in this leadership position for over a decade. This third "name" for the organization lasted until 1932 when the organization enfolded some of the additional public health services offered by the Red Cross; it then became known as Public Health Nursing and Home Hygiene and Care of the Sick.

In the early 1920s the organization experienced for a short time an increase in the number of chapters. Soon after, the numbers declined as many of these chapters were unable to be successful in their own operations. The ARC chapters faced competition from the many tax-supported agencies, tuberculosis associations, other voluntary health agencies, and professional groups that also provided some public health nursing services.[40] Even within the organization, nursing staff members questioned some of the work being done by the Red Cross. Mabel Boardman, one of the early proponents of Town and Country, found herself embroiled in a disagreement over the Central Committee's new direction of assuming a broader responsibility for the health of the country.[41] Mary Beard also spoke against the plan for expansion of public health services directed from the top. Instead she said expansion should come from within the community and "develop slowly, with local understanding and support."[42]

Insufficient Number of Qualified Rural Public Health Nurses

In addition to her concerns over expansion, Mary Beard was also concerned about the lack of qualified rural public health nurses. In a presentation to the 29th Annual Meeting of the National League of Nursing Education, Beard responded to the Rockefeller Report Analysis of the Situation in the Public Health Field. Known as the Goldmark Report, the report presented what many in the profession, especially those in the rural nursing service, already knew—there were not a sufficient number of public health nurses to provide the communities around the country with the preventive and bedside care that was needed. In 1923, Beard explained:

> Miss Goldmark's concise language making it perfectly clear what is meant, that, while the life of the public health nurse is an intensely absorbing and attractive one, it has not yet made a sufficiently strong

appeal to the kind of young people needed to supply the 85,000 public health nurses needed in the United States. There are 12,000 and we need 85,000![43]

ARC historian Portia Kernodle wrote that the "decade of the 1930s was a bad time for the Red Cross Nursing Service," just as it was for every other agency. Throughout the depression, the Red Cross Nursing Service "fought not only disease but poverty and despair."[44] The leadership of the ARC changed when Fox resigned in 1930 and Malinde Havey became the National Director of the Public Health Nursing Service. Her role in the organization continued to grow as the service expanded in 1932 to include the Red Cross's other public health role in the community, the Home Hygiene and Care of the Sick Division. Havey remained in that position until her death in 1938. During the remaining 10 years that the service existed, a series of nursing leaders assumed that leadership position, finally culminating with Mary Beard as the final leader. These leaders continually faced the problems created by economic constraints, Roosevelt's new federal social legislation, and the uncertainty shared by the rest of the country.[45]

"Poverty and misery somehow focus[ed] on the doorstep of the public health nurse," wrote Havey. Public health nurses simultaneously faced difficulty in financing their local services while experiencing an increased demand in these services. Havey was concerned that public health nurses were becoming more engaged in "charity work" than in nursing.[46] In 1932, after surveying all Red Cross chapters, the leadership decided the unification of the Public Health Nursing Services with the Home Hygiene and Care of the Sick was necessary.

At about the same time, President Roosevelt's "New Deal" legislation created the Federal Emergency Relief Administration (1932) and the Civil Works Administration (1933). These federal organizations began to fund the work of nurses in public health and home hygiene. This funding significantly increased the number of participants in the home hygiene classroom program, thus creating challenges for the ARC to find enough settings in which to provide those classes. With an overabundance of unemployed nurses, the Red Cross was inundated with applicants for the home hygiene program. Now they faced the task of assuring that every nurse was qualified. Training of the newly hired nurses in the skills needed to teach these classes became a necessary part of the nursing service. Additional funding came from other areas as well to accommodate the expanding role of the public health nursing service to provide instruction to mothers. The increase in funding sources "bolstered the morale of communities" and the Red Cross staff as well.[47]

Since the Social Security Act of the 1930s also increased the amount of funds available for nursing services, more nurses elected to work in public health agencies rather than in private voluntary agencies. Voluntary agencies such as the Red Cross continued to be seen as a healthy competitor to the official agencies, but their role in public health nursing was losing ground. With the funds received from the new Social Security Act, the United States Public Health service established its own nursing division in 1935 to find ways to employ over six thousand unemployed nurses. This nursing division grew in strength in the next few years as it experienced a strong following in the nursing community. This new direction for nursing added another blow to the declining role of the ARC public health nursing service.[48]

The many reports of the 1930s showed a decline in the ARC services, difficulty with relationships in communities, and difficulty in meeting the needs of the community for public health nursing services. During this period the NOPHN examined the relationship of the ARC and public health nursing, and recommended that more "emphasis [be] placed on working with state health departments and on transferring services to other agencies whenever possible."[49] Mary Beard also questioned the Red Cross's ability to provide quality public health nursing services, because in her view many of the "local Chapters and Committees [were] not well informed [nor] closely in touch with professional ideals."[50] As a result of the many structural changes, Alta Dines, who led one of the studies, wrote in a 1938 report that the "American Red Cross had lost its position of leadership in nursing."[51] Dines recommended that public health nurses return to the "remote areas [that] state departments of health could not reach, doing pioneer work in demonstration."[52] It was a suggestion to revert back to the original concept of the ARC rural nursing service rather than continue their expanded efforts assumed since the late 1920s. However, with America's entrance into World War II, the public health nursing service again changed as the war effort became the Red Cross's main focus.

CONCLUDING YEARS OF THE ARC RURAL
PUBLIC HEALTH NURSING SERVICE

By 1942, a decline in rural public health services was seen as a direct result of the increased demands for nurses in World War II. Elisabeth Vaughn, the National Director of Public Health Nursing at the time, was concerned about the loss of standards that typified the ARC since its inception and wanted services to close rather than provide inferior care. The closure of these services was waylaid, however, by the efforts of the Metropolitan Life Insurance Company that continued to hold policyholder contracts with the ARC. Rather than have the ARC shut down the services immediately, Metropolitan Life preferred a "gradual" closure of the ARC's services to "allow communities time to develop necessary local organization to continue service."[53] In response, the ARC established a Special Medical and Health Survey Committee to review the status of the existing rural public health service. They studied the many criticisms directed at the service since 1939 and found that the concerns of the many years of controversy were mounting rather than dissipating. They recommended the end of the Red Cross's involvement in local public health nursing and supported the idea of public health services fitting under one "general plan sponsored by an official agency."[54] By December 1947, the ARC Board of Governors approved the recommendations of the Committee on Nursing of the Advisory Board on Health Services: ". . . the Red Cross should discontinue its existing local public health nursing services."[55] This meant that the one hundred remaining local public health nursing services would be transferred to other agencies in the community or closed by June 30, 1950. The two hundred public health nurses employed by those local chapters would be transferred or should seek employment elsewhere.

Thus, the Town and Country Service, begun in 1912, ended in 1947 after several long years of decline in funding, lack of qualified nursing staff, increasing community resistance, and competitive response from various organizations, including those within the profession.[56] These nurses had served in an exciting and innovative organization that used the existing organizational structure of the ARC to develop a national network that provided public health nurses to rural communities and towns throughout the United States. Although this service promised a way to distribute rural health services to those in need throughout the nation, it faced challenges throughout its history that eventually led to its demise. Criticism often focused on the placement of public health nurses in communities by the ARC rather than from within the communities themselves; the ever-increasing competition from official public health agencies, voluntary organizations, and private practitioners in the community; and the ability to meet the standards set by the organization.[57] Yet the very focus on rural health by many nursing leaders during the early part of the 20th century illustrates the necessity for this kind of nursing service and the need for adequately educated professionals to carry on this work with a "most earnest purpose" and a "deep sense of spirit."[58]

CONCLUSION

Despite the many challenges that the rural public health nursing program faced throughout the years, the fact remains that between 1913 and 1947, there were over "3,109 public health nursing services in about 1,800 counties under the sponsorship of some 2,100 chapters—a notable contribution to the health of America and an influence on many other agencies."[59]

The ARC's foray into peacetime rural public health nursing services and the requirement for nurses to receive additional education in public health to participate in these services supported the profession's effort to raise standards of nursing education. Since the ARC required advanced education and found ways to offer scholarships and loans to students, many postgraduate programs in public health nursing emerged, with Teachers College at the forefront. Rural health care influenced the development of these advanced programs in public health nursing and raised the level of awareness that nurses needed to learn more than what was offered in a basic diploma program. Nurses needed to be accomplished in bedside care as well as in health promotion and disease prevention activities to meet the needs of rural communities across America.

Although public health nurses may never have successfully developed the "kind of organizational structures that might have permitted them to be a cohesive, recognized, and powerful group"[60] (as some historians have suggested), we can learn other lessons from the work of these ARC rural public health nurses. The needs of those living in rural counties and smaller towns across America continue to remain a concern for health care providers. It was the work of nurses that made this a successful venture in most cases.[61] Regardless of the tensions surrounding the supply of public health nurses to rural communities, the work of public health nurses provided all aspects of public health nursing services to populations that typically did not receive service. It was their ability to meet ARC standards, provide care to communities while facing all kinds of barriers, and yet still be able to be a group that showed a "most earnest purpose, a deep spirit of service."[62]

NOTES

1. Lillian Wald to Jacob Schiff in 1910 cited in Lavinia L. Dock, Sarah E. Pickett, Fannie F. Clement, Elizabeth G. Fox, and Anna R. Van Meter, *History of American Red Cross Nursing* (New York, NY: Macmillan, 1922), 1213.

2. Dock, *History of American Red Cross Nursing*, 1213.

3. Dock, *History of American Red Cross Nursing*, 1213.

4. Dock, *History of American Red Cross Nursing*, 1213.

5. Dock, *History of American Red Cross Nursing*, 1216.

6. Requirements for the candidates to the ARC included: "minimum age of twenty-five, a doctor's certificate with renewal every two years, and a certificate of registration in states where registration was required and in other states graduate from a recognized school of nursing with a course of not less than two years." See Portia B. Kernodle, *The Red Cross Nurse in Action 1882–1948* (New York, NY: Harper & Brothers, 1949), 43.

7. Minutes of the Second Meeting of the Committee on Rural Nursing, December 10, 1912: p. 1. (Rockefeller Sanitary Commission Microfilm, Reel 1, Folder 8, ARC Town and Country Nursing Service 1912–1914).

8. To assure the quality of the nurses, they established scholarships and loans that would help nurses fulfill the requirement needed to join this service.

9. Minutes of the Third Meeting of the Committee on Rural Nursing, May 5, 1913, p. 2. (Rockefeller Sanitary Commission Microfilm, Reel 1, Folder 8, ARC Town and Country Nursing Service 1912–1914). Even the size of a rural community was specified by the Committee in their literature by using the classification of cities by the United States. Five thousand was the suggested maximum population in a "rural" community.

10. ARC Rural Nursing Service, Circular for Application, Rockefeller Sanitary Commission Microfilm, Reel 1, Folder 8, ARC Town and Country Nursing Service 1912–1914.

11. Mabel Boardman, letter to Mr. Wickliff Rose, Rockefeller Sanitary Commission Microfilm, Reel 1, Folder 8, ARC Town and Country Nursing Service 1912–1914, May 21, 1913.

12. Mr. Wickliff Rose, letter to Miss Mabel Boardman, Rockefeller Sanitary Commission Microfilm, Reel 1, Folder 8, ARC Town and Country Nursing Service 1912–1914, May 30, 1913.

13. Suggestions for the Organization of a Local Nursing Association, Rockefeller Sanitary Commission Microfilm, Reel 1, Folder 8, ARC Town and Country Nursing Service 1912–1914.

14. Suggested Duties of a Local Organization, Rockefeller Sanitary Commission Microfilm, Reel 1, Folder 8, ARC Town and Country Nursing Service 1912–1914.

15. Elizabeth Fox, "Red Cross Public Health Nursing, Out to Sea," *Public Health Nurse* 13 (1921): 105–108 (found digitalized by Google) (quote, p. 105).

16. Fox, "Red Cross Public Health Nursing, Out to Sea," 105.

17. Regulations for Rural Nurses Appointed by the Red Cross, Rockefeller Sanitary Commission Microfilm, Reel 1, Folder 8, ARC Town and Country Nursing Service 1912–1914.

18. Fannie Clement, "Town and Country Nursing Service," *American Journal of Nursing* 16, no. 11 (1916): 1117–120 (quote, p. 1120).

19. Fox, "Red Cross Nursing," 105.

20. Fox, "Red Cross Nursing," 105.

21. Fox, "Red Cross Nursing," 105.

22. Fox, "Red Cross Nursing," 108.

23. Post Graduate Courses for Red Cross Town and Country Nursing Service Candidates (four months course), 1914–1915, Pocket Knowledge, Department of Nursing and Health, American Red Cross Town and Country Nursing Service, published 1899–1961, uploaded 6/15/2009 by Pocket Masters, Archives of the Department of Nursing Education, 0397.pdf file, p. 2.

24. "Post Graduate Courses for Red Cross Town and Country Nursing Service Candidates (four months course), 1914–1915."

25. Lillian Wald cited in Dock et al., *History of American Red Cross Nursing* (1922), 1214.

26. The ARC Rural Nursing Service, Scope, third bullet point, Rockefeller Sanitary Commission Microfilm, Reel 1, Folder 8, ARC Town and Country Nursing Service 1912–1914.

27. Suggestions for the Organization of a Local Nursing Association, Rockefeller Sanitary Commission Microfilm, Reel 1, Folder 8, ARC Town and Country Nursing Service 1912–1914.

28. Suggestions for the Organization of a Local Nursing Association, Rockefeller Sanitary Commission Microfilm, Reel 1, Folder 8, ARC Town and Country Nursing Service 1912–1914.

29. Minutes of the Fourth Meeting of the Committee on Rural Nursing, October 22, 1913, p. 1. (Rockefeller Sanitary Commission Microfilm, Reel 1, Folder 8, ARC Town and Country Nursing Service 1912–1914).

30. Dock, *History of American Red Cross Nursing* (1922), 1218.

31. Elizabeth G. Fox, "Twenty Years of Red Cross Public Health Nursing," *The Red Cross Courier*, 12, no. 6 (December 1932): 173–175 (quote, p. 173).

32. Fox, "Twenty Years of Red Cross Public Health Nursing," 173.

33. Fox, "Twenty Years of Red Cross Public Health Nursing," 173.

34. Minutes of the Fourth Meeting of the Committee on Red Cross Rural Nursing, October 22, 1913 (Rockefeller Sanitary Commission Microfilm, Reel 1, Folder 8, ARC Town and Country Nursing Service 1912–1914).

35. Mary Roberts, *American Nursing: History and Interpretation* (New York, NY: MacMillan, 1954).

36. Minutes of the Fifth Meeting of the Committee on Town and Country Nursing, December 9, 1913, p. 1 (Rockefeller Sanitary Commission Microfilm, Reel 1, Folder 8, ARC Town and Country Nursing Service 1912–1914); Dock et al. *History of American Red Cross Nursing* (1922), 1220–221.

37. Fox, "Twenty Years of Red Cross Public Health Nursing," 174.

38. Roberts, *American Nursing*.

39. Dock et al., *History of American Red Cross Nursing*, 1274. For discussion about Gardner's work in Italy, see Dock, et al. *History of American Red Cross Nursing* (1922), 867–69.

40. Portia Kernodle, *The Red Cross Nurse in Action 1882–1948* (New York, NY: Harper and Brothers, 1949), 275.

41. Kernodle, *The Red Cross Nurse in Action 1882–1948*, 276.

42. Kernodle, *The Red Cross Nurse in Action 1882–1948*, 275.

43. Mary Beard, "Analysis of Situation in Public Health Field, Discussion of the Rockefeller Report Analysis of the Situation in the Public Health Field," *Twenty-ninth*

Annual Report of the National League of Nursing Education, (Baltimore, MD: Williams & Wilkins, 1923), 180.

44. Kernodle, *The Red Cross,* 360.

45. Kernodle, *The Red Cross,* 362–63.

46. Kernodle, *The Red Cross,* 363.

47. Kernodle, *The Red Cross,* 369.

48. Kernodle, *The Red Cross,* 377.

49. Kernodle, *The Red Cross,* 380.

50. Mary Beard in Kernodle, *The Red Cross,* 380.

51. Mary Beard in Kernodle, *The Red Cross,* 373.

52. Mary Beard in Kernodle, *The Red Cross,* 380.

53. Mary Beard in Kernodle, *The Red Cross,* 468.

54. Mary Beard in Kernodle, *The Red Cross,* 468.

55. Mary Beard in Kernodle, *The Red Cross,* 469.

56. Town and Country was the second name assigned to the ARC Rural Nursing Service; it was not the last. The name changed several times throughout its existence and each time the change represented the broadening of responsibilities assumed by the ARC in providing public health nursing. See Table 1 for the changing names and the reasons for those changes.

57. Portia Kernodle, *The Red Cross Nurse in Action 1882–1948* (New York, NY: Harper and Brothers, 1949); Jerri L. Bigbee and Eleanor L. M. Crowder, "The Red Cross Rural Nursing Service: An Innovative Model of Public Health Nursing Delivery," *Public Health Nursing* 2, no. 2 (1985): 109–21; Karen Buhler-Wilkerson, *False Dawn: The Rise and Decline of Public Health Nursing, 1900–1930* (New York, NY: Garland, 1989).

58. Fannie F. Clement, "Town and Country Nursing Service," *American Journal of Nursing* 16, no. 11 (1916): 1117–120 (quote, p. 1120).

59. Kernodle, *The Red Cross,* 469.

60. Karen Buhler-Wilkerson, "Bringing Care to the People: Lillian Wald's Legacy to Public Health Nursing," *American Journal of Public Health,* 83, no. 12 (1993): 1778–786 (quote, p. 1783).

61. Kernodle, *The Red Cross,* 469.

62. Clement, "Town and Country Nursing Service," 1120.

2

•••••

Public Nursing in Rural Wisconsin: Stretched Beyond Health Instruction

•••••

RIMA D. APPLE

"AM SORRY I CANNOT BE IN TWO PLACES AT ONCE" admitted Teresa Gardner in November of 1922, a claim she probably uttered frequently during her career as county nurse of Price County, Wisconsin.[1] Many public health nurses through the century have undoubtedly muttered similar sentiments about their varied, complex, labor-intensive, and time-consuming work. The experiences of Gardner and her predecessor Ernestine Kandel, however, are unique. Rural public health was slowly emerging in the early 20th century. The field itself lacked a clear definition and its practitioners worked in environments dominated by the poverty and the isolation of widely dispersed farms, villages, and small towns. The critical need for health education, nursing care, and preventive medicine in the areas outside urban United States was evident. With few rural cities large enough to sustain a public health department, the Wisconsin State Department of Health decided to appoint public health nurses on the county level as an effective way to bring the benefits of modern medicine to an extremely underserved population. The goals were clear, yet the path to those goals was not. Studying the professional lives of the public health nurses of rural Wisconsin highlights their successes and their problems and, in so doing, enables us to better understand the multiplicity of elements that shaped the struggle for public health in the rural United States.

THE FIRST COUNTY NURSES

The 1913 state statutes first defined the role of county nurse in Wisconsin. The nurse was to be a trained graduate nurse, responsible for examining school children not examined by a visiting nurse or physician; to assist the county superintendent of the poor; to identify and instruct tuberculosis patients; and to act "as visiting nurse throughout the county to perform such other duties as nurse and hygienic expert as may be assigned to her by the county board." She was to document her work in a monthly report to the county board in which she "shall show the visits made during the month ending and the requests made to her for services, and such other information as the county board may from time to time require."[2] The statute created the position of county nurse, but apparently few counties had the finances or the will to appoint one in this period. The situation changed in 1919 when Wisconsin mandated the appointment of county nurses, though the state still provided no funding for the position. These nurses were to supervise children in school; assist the "superintendent of the poor"; identify, report, and treat cases of tuberculosis; investigate cases of child neglect and delinquency; assist in investigating cases of truancy, child labor, and crippled children; and "to act as health instructor throughout the county and to perform such other duties as may be assigned to her."[3] By meeting these role expectations, the county nurse was both a health worker and a social worker.

Shortly before the law made the employment of county nurses compulsory, Price County hired Ernestine Kandel for the position. At this time, Price County was one of the few counties in Wisconsin to make such an appointment.[4] Kandel left in the fall of 1921, at which time she was succeeded by Teresa Gardner. Both women were avid proponents of public health efforts and the role of the public health nurse. They willingly and eagerly took on the many and varied roles assigned to them, and expanded their activities to improve the health and the material and social conditions of the county's population. Their work was greatly appreciated by the residents. And yet, in 1924, the county abolished the position of county nurse. Kandel's and Gardner's experiences in Price County point to the problems that had plagued and could have defeated any early public health efforts in the rural United States.

Price County is located in far northern Wisconsin, a rectangle 31 miles wide and 42 miles long, making it one of the largest counties in the state. Gardner found the distances both exhausting and exhilarating, remarking, "Frequently I drive 15 to 75 miles a day and occassionly [sic] 100 to 125 and the work left undone would be nerve [sic] racking if I did not have the fresh air and beautiful green fields or snow banks to counteract and stimulate."[5] In the 19th and early 20th centuries, the lumber industry dominated the county's economy. As the pine forests were depleted, farming became more common, though the poor soil limited its success. In the 1910s and 1920s, the dying lumber industry resulted in stressed financial conditions and a struggling population of lumberjacks and farmers, many of whom were immigrants to the United States. Consequently, the definition of the county nurse as both a health worker and a social worker placed Kandel and Gardner in a challenging position: how to fulfill these two needed and demanding roles.

DEFINING THE WORK OF THE COUNTY NURSE

Kandel's first monthly report documents the hectic pace in the office.[6] She began on August 20, 1919, by reviewing the county's vital statistics and "found a very high infant mortality rate, even after making allowances for faulty registration." She then "called on County Officials, Doctors, Clergy, and heads of the various departments of the Red Cross." Over the remainder of the month, she held "mothers meetings" in five communities, during which she explained "school inspection and the results expected from it. Also explained the many other uses they [the mothers] might have for the help of the County Nurse." At each school she inspected the children and often found problems such as "defective teeth," "defective hearing (running ear)," "enlarged glands of neck," and "very backward in school work/ has defective nasal breathing, defective hearing, and vision." She wrote to the parents of each of these children, advising that they see a doctor for further examination.[7] At each of the schools she also organized Health Crusader Clubs.[8] The National Tuberculosis Association designed this program to instill in children good health habits, such as brushing teeth, bathing, sleeping with the window open, and drinking three glasses of water a day, but no tea or coffee. The county nurse worked with teachers to set up the program and instructed the students to record their activities on grade sheets that provided the basis for awards at the end of the contest. Kandel considered this education of children one of the most critical aspects of her work, asserting:

> the good derived from the Modern Health Crusade work in the school would in itself justify the existence of a county nurse, if she did nothing more than see that every child was enrolled and carried out the rules daily.[9]

Kandel's work was not limited to the schools. In the same few weeks in August 1919, she also visited the town of Lugerville, the site of "a great many cases of whooping cough," where she informed the residents of the "importance of preventing the futher [sic] spread of the disease." Four of the homes she saw were "very unclean" and several had sick children who had not seen a doctor. When she returned to the town a few days later, she learned "that the doctor had not been called out but a decided improvement in cleanliness was observed in one case." She also visited several others: an expectant mother whom she advised, the family of a delinquent girl, and four soldiers who had returned from the hospital and needed information about the government insurance program. In addition, she called on all the doctors and dentists in the neighboring towns. Kandel also followed tuberculosis patients who had returned from the General Hospital and attempted to get these patients admitted to the tuberculosis sanatorium. She also wrote 14 business letters.[10] Her October report documents similar activities; she reported dealing with one case of measles, one suspected case of smallpox, and eight cases of diphtheria, which she happily noted were "not severe, as all cases had serum after discovery of first case–contacts examined." In January 1921 her additional tasks included arranging quarantines for cases of diphtheria and other infectious diseases, transporting patients to sanitaria, and lecturing teachers and students in the normal school. This pace continued through the ensuing months as she visited more schools to examine students and identify "defects," held more mothers meetings, wrote innumerable letters, supervised the rest tent at the county fair, advocated for hot school lunches, transported children to the hospital for tonsillectomies, visited homes, and held office hours.[11]

This county nurse did not limit her activities to health and health instruction, however. Kandel's descriptions of home visits are useful examples of how her health work and social work were entwined. In September of 1919, she returned to Lugerville to follow up on the cases of whooping cough she had found the previous month. "Children now having medical attention and one showing marked improvement," she happily wrote. However, all was not well in the town. A "second child altho [sic] having medical attention is neglected at home, where a fourteen year old girl is taking care of a family of five." Kandel optimistically reported that she "Will try to better the social conditions."[12] In another case,

> Called at Home of Indigent family. Father with frozen toe—Sent to hospital[.] Toe amputated. Cases [sic] reported to Insurance Company by employer as not having sufficient stockings on—Refused insurance. Chairman of County Board looking matter up. Clothing supplied.[13]

In this instance, Kandel could not separate the medical concerns from the social conditions under which her patient was living. Given the poverty of the area, it is likely that the patient could not afford appropriate footwear, a factor that the insurance company disregarded but Kandel could not. Moreover, her social work was not always a sideline of her health work. Her reports are full of cases such as in January 1921 when she informed a father that his "incorrigable" [sic] daughter was being returned home after a short jail sentence. Acting more as a parole officer than a nurse, Kandel informed the girl and her family "that girl would be sent to State Institution at first indiscretion."[14] In another instance, to improve the home conditions of nine neglected children, she found a housekeeper and the "Court gave me custody of [the] children."

Her professional scope was stretched even beyond health instruction, and soldiers, and poor housekeeping, and "incorrigible" girls to community interests such as Americanization classes, Civic League meetings, and publicity for a tuberculosis clinic. For instance, in the month of October she had to arrange food and clothing for three families on relief and "Two housekeepers installed in families where girls under fourteen years of age were caring for large families." Typical of her social work, in January of 1920 she made two calls in the town of Catawba to investigate the need for state aid, and determined in each case to award $20 per month. She would follow up on such calls to judge whether the amount was sufficient.

When Gardner succeeded Kandel in 1921, she continued these wide-ranging activities with energy and fervor, reflecting both her personal enthusiasm and that of the county's population. Her lengthy letter to Mary R. Morgan, Director of the Wisconsin Bureau of Child Welfare and Public Health Nursing, clearly conveys her pleasure in this work and the importance of community to her health work.

I am writing you the day after the first conference with mothers as I know you are interested in the outcome of it. We had a conference at Pennington and the women have a Community Club that meets monthly, occasionally meeting in the evening with the husbands present. Yesterday there were twenty-four women present and during the noon hour four or five of their husbands dropped in for lunch. There were fourteen children under school age who were brought in to be weighed and measured. This included all but two of the children in the district. Two of these children were decidedly underweight. Questioning one mother I found that they had no cow and the child was not having milk at all. An elderly woman spoke up at once and said the woman could send over and have a quart or two of milk every day for her children. This woman lived on the adjoining farm a distance of half a mile and the offer was accepted. I feel one remedy will be applied immediately towards the building up of that child.

It was an enthusiastic meeting and the women were very appreciative . . . I had posters from the national Child Welfare Association, the set of six, "Aids for the Nutritional Clinic," eight Mother Goose Health Rhymes, and some posters from the Makers of American Ideals and the American Citizen and Early Habit Forming. Also a complete model infant[']s layette, using these posters as illustrative material, followed by discussion. The conference lasted from 10:30 a.m. till 4 p.m., including two luncheons. It closed . . . with reading from the Bible and Prayer.

The community has always interested me. Although they are made up of several nationalities, a few well educated people and some foreigners who cannot understand English, they cooperate and work together for the common good and have really accomplished a great deal within the last three years.[15]

At meetings such as these Gardner weighed and measured preschool children, alerted parents (usually mothers) to potential health problems with their children, and instructed both mothers and children in appropriate health routines. Gardner, though in an isolated rural area, was acutely aware of public health efforts outside the county and utilized educational material developed by national organizations. Her detailed description demonstrates the flexibility of mothers meetings and the potential for unintended consequences. One unplanned aspect of such an event was that fathers attended part of the meeting, though it is not clear if they came for the education or the food. Another and perhaps more critical outcome was the connection made between neighbors in order to ameliorate a family's problem. The neighboring farms were only a half mile apart, but it was the meeting that alerted one neighbor to the plight of the other.

From this and other reports sent back to Morgan, Gardner clearly delighted in the instructional aspect of her job. In addition to mothers meetings, she organized an educational tent at the County Fair and she particularly enjoyed teaching Little Mothers classes, in which girls were taught appropriate, usually middle-class childcare techniques.[16] Health educators and public health officials believed that such classes were necessary especially for the poor, both rural and urban, in whose families both parents worked outside the home and the younger children were left in the care of their slightly older siblings. Kandel, and later Gardner, found many families attended by a teenager who handled most of the daily childcare routines. Sometimes it was possible to bring a housekeeper into the home, but that could be expensive for the family or the county. Alternatively, training girls in proper techniques would enable them to better care for their sisters and brothers and also prepare them for motherhood. Gardner devoted much of June 1924 to Little Mothers classes, to such an extent that she limited her other work, "doing," in her words, "only the necessary Social Service work."

> My first class was at 8:30 in the morning in Phillips. Classes usually were an hour to an hour and a quarter. Then I drove 12 miles to Lugerville. We had a class from 10:30 to 11:45, then I drove 8 miles to Fifield, where we had a class from 1 to 2:30. I then drove 6 miles to Park Falls and we held a class from 3 to 4:30, returning to Philips, a distance of 20 miles. The equipment being carried in a blue denim bag, but the enthusiasm of the children has more than paid for the labor expended. . . ."[17]

Forty-six miles each day on rural roads represents Gardner's commitment to health education.

Though she spent many hours in instructional work, Gardner, like Kandel, found herself in the midst of complicated family issues that tangled health and social work. A dramatic and telling example of this is the case of H. R. In June of 1923, W. J. M., of Ogema, Wisconsin, sent a letter to Gardner informing her that a neighbor girl, H. R., "[gets] the fits every day and she is asking for help."[18] W. J. M. also wrote the county judge about the case and requested that the nurse visit the girl. Gardner did so and found that H. R. was "shy—hair uncombed—dress dirty—house dirty."[19] H. R. admitted that she had "spells six or eight times a day" and Gardner described the treatment the girl had undergone:

> Dr. Miller has helped her. She has taken a number of bottles of Nervine.[20] Has had spells three years she says. Had all her teeth extracted and tonsils taken out but it did not help her.[21]

Gardner also spoke with one of H. R.'s brothers-in-law, who echoed the worries of W. J. M. and insisted that the girl should be institutionalized. The next day Gardner continued her investigation, visiting a half-sister of H. R. in Prentice, Wisconsin. She learned that the husband of this woman was so concerned about the situation that he "asked a year ago for an application blank to fill out to put her in an institution." Ultimately nothing was done because, as the nurse explained, "the family opposed it."[22]

Gardner was in the middle of a family disagreement over the appropriate treatment for H. R.'s "fits." The record does not show if the nurse contacted the physician at this time. However, a few days later, Gardner received a letter that clarified who objected to the institutionalization, though not why. The plaintive and confused note, written in a childish hand, came from H. R. herself, pleading:

> I must let you know that I am not going there where you were going to take me pa said he wont sign the papers he don't want me to so you don't have to bother any more if I can't come back any pa told me I would have to stay there all the time I couldn't come home any more.[23]

Whether this letter deterred Gardner from further action or if the nurse was distracted by her many other and perhaps more immediate tasks is not revealed in the record. But the case, as with a number of the cases, disappeared only to reappear months later. In early November, when at the Liberty School in Ogema examining students, Gardner inquired about H. R.'s family and learned that in the summer the father, who had so strenuously objected to placing his daughter in an institution, had fallen from a hay stack and died. Subsequently H. R. had moved in with her half-sister and her husband in Prentice; the same couple who had earlier considered placing H. R. in an institution. A few weeks later, Gardner learned that H. R. and a younger brother were now living with a different family. Gardner's records do not document the steps she took next, but the last line of her case notes, dated November 28, 1923, reads: "[H. R.] committed to the home for the feeble minded at Chippewa Falls."[24] The outline of this case documents the multiple facets of the work of a public health nurse in rural, poverty-stricken Wisconsin in the 1920s. Other mandated tasks, such as school inspections and the follow-up of contagious diseases, limited the time that Gardner could spend on cases that did not demand immediate attention.

The work of the Wisconsin county nurse was extremely complex and both Kandel and Gardner saw need and often sought solutions. Their interest in the health and welfare of the county led them to expand their roles. They wrote letters and visited homes "to let people hnow [sic] in what way I can be of service to them."[25] They pushed the county board to provide hot lunches in schools, and encouraged the Commercial Club of Park Falls to open its membership to boys and young men so they could use the club two nights a week.[26]

Possibly the most significant factor complicating the work of the county nurse was the sheer number of people who could and did call upon her services. She had little control over her own time. In the case of H. R., Gardner received direction or prodding from a judge and a concerned neighbor, and Morgan prompted her to offer Little Mothers classes. County nurses also received instructions from the county board members. Residents like

Mrs. O. W. H. wrote letters anticipating that the nurse could and would answer her many questions, including:

> advise me when I should begin to wean my baby. He is nearly 13 Months now.
> Nights when he is asleep he has cold sweat spells. gets them some times during the day. He has 8 teeth so far.
> I am preant [sic] again, I have not menstruation [sic] for over three months.
> I am bothered with morning sickness and am very weeks [sic] also. Hopeing [sic] you can advise me what is best to do.[27]

Other requests were less specific. Gardner visited Mrs. R., who wrote that she had "something I would like to consult with you about." The county nurse expected a conversation about Mrs. R's daughter who had recently recovered from pneumonia. Instead:

> It was simply gossip in regard to her neighbors that she wished to see me about. Told her hereafter that I would not call at her request unless she states in her letter what she wished to see me about.[28]

Obviously, some clients were more interested in sociality than health care. Other residents gave nurses "many helpful hints as to people who needed help from" the county nurse.[29] Still others wrote letters of thanks to "My dear friend."[30] Teachers called upon the county nurses to supervise the national Modern Health Crusade and examine students, and alerted them to possible cases of contagious diseases, which had to be investigated. Local health officers directed county nurses to placard houses when necessary. The state Bureau of Communicable Diseases asked that nurses check the weekly report of cases of communicable disease for accuracy and inform of any changes. Then there were also the local physicians.

NURSE–PHYSICIAN RELATIONSHIPS

As a nurse entered a county, one of her first tasks was to speak with each of the local physicians; to assure him (in Price County at this time all the physicians were male) that she was there to support his work, not replace him; and to ask him to sign or amend her standing orders. The State Board of Health insisted on this practice for practical and professional reasons. Each physician who personally evaluated the standing orders "might have some little changes which he wanted to make and which can be made on the copy

which he signs." Being involved in the defining of the standing orders ensured that the physician did not feel that the nurse or the state was directing
his practice.[31] It also established a hierarchy in which the nurse was sub-
ordinate to the doctor and, Mary P. Morgan, the Director of the Bureau of
Child Welfare and Public Health Nursing insisted, "a definite understanding
of the subject of giving or recommending treatment will protect you [the
nurse] from possible criticism."[32] Some physicians did make alterations to
the standing orders, but most did not; the majority of local physicians signed
and then utilized the nurses in their work.

The nurse–physician relationship had many dimensions. When the
nurses examined school children and found "defects," or when they visited
homes where they discovered a pregnant woman or an ill child who had not
been seen by a physician, they directed the client to see the local physician.
A physician might notice a potential outbreak of a contagious disease and
notify the nurse of the risk so that she could investigate further. F. W. Mitchell,
MD, of Ogema, Wisconsin, wrote Gardner in December of 1921 with the
information that he had visited a 5-year-old with the symptoms of scarlet
fever and had heard rumors of other children who had been sick and missed
school. He recommended "that it would be a good plan for you to run down
if you can tomorrow and look at this school."[33] Similarly, when the nurse
saw a questionable case, she would ask the family to call in the physician to
confirm the situation. When Gardner visited Park Falls on January 27, 1922,
some of the teachers told her that they suspected an "outbreak of scarlet
fever" because they had observed possible symptoms on some of the children in one room. Gardner wrote to inform the local physician and offered
that "if this report is not exaggerated would you like my assistance in examining the pupils?" She admitted that she would need to change her schedule.
She was not planning on returning to Park Falls until late in February, but
she could come earlier to weigh and measure, and make the "yearly examination of the school of Park Falls."[34]

THE REALITY OF BUDGETARY CONSTRAINTS

Considering the extensive public health and social work conducted by Kandel
and Gardner, and the accolades they received from the community, the position of county nurse in Price County would seem to be secure. However, not
everyone saw the situation that way. Over the years of their tenure, Kandel
and Gardner faced several challenges; most often it was financial factors,
not their activities, that contributed to the struggle to maintain the position.
Within a year of Kandel's appointment, she had won the approval of many
in the county. The County Health Committee proudly reported that the

county nurse "shows the importance of this public health work." Its testimonial to her included a recommendation that the county employ an additional nurse.[35] However, the county board did not concur. The request for a second nurse was renewed the next year, to no avail, though with a hopeful sign. "I was really surprised when the request of a second nurse ended in a tie at the last board meeting," Kandel reported to Morgan, "as in the face of the present unrest that was much more than I expected, and was really in doubt as to whether we should have the matter brought up at all at this time."[36] It is not clear what Kandel meant by "unrest." It is likely that since she had announced that she would be leaving Price County a few months later, the county board wanted to see her replacement before making the decision to hire another nurse.

A serious threat to the position itself occurred 2 years later. One of the county supervisors recommended that the nurse's salary be reduced. Ignoring the many different efforts of the county nurse, he considered that "the main part of the work of the County Nurse of Price County is and should be devoted to the inspection of the school children." He calculated from Gardner's annual report that she had spent 351 hours, or 58.5 school days, examining students, and concluded that her $2,000 salary was "not believed to be commensurate with the benefits received." At the May 1923 board meeting, he submitted a resolution to reduce the salary to $1,000, with another $1,000 in an expense allowance.[37] The motion was passed on a vote of 23 to three.[38] Gardner had vocal allies in the community, particularly among local women's groups, notably the Woman's Christian Temperance Union of the town of Phillips and the St. Margaret's Guild, which came to her defense. Considering "the law establishing a County Nurse as one of the most humane of our legislature," stressing the importance of caring for "the poor, needy, and often illiterate of our people [as] the wisest for our economy," praising Gardner "for her very efficient work in all departments of her office," and concluding that such a position should be "adequately recompensed," they petitioned the board to reconsider its vote.[39]

Gardner answered as well in two extensive articles in local newspapers. In one, she detailed the diverse aspects of her role in supporting the health and welfare of the county. In the other, rather than correcting the mistaken idea that her work was focused on school examinations, she instead focused on economics. In her open letter to the "taxpayers" of the county, published in the *Phillips Times* of June 2, 1923, she alerted the community to an aspect of her position they may not have been aware of, which, she pointed out, had saved tax dollars.

Your school tax is high and rightly so.
You have a large amount of money invested in schools.

If schools are closed on account of contagion, the teacher's salary continues and she is not required to make up the time, the pupils lose time that cannot be made up and the equipment is idle.

The county nurse has on request inspected schools for contagion in the following towns and assisted in establishing quarantine, and with only a few exceptions the schools have remained open with no spread of the disease in the communities where the quarantine rules have been conscientiously observed.

Then she listed fifteen school districts that she had inspected.[40] Gardner justified the position of county nurse not because public health efforts were good for the community and its residents, but because it saved money.

This was a potent argument in 1923. The previous year the county supervisors had asked the state legislature to alter the county nurse statute "so that the same shall apply only to such counties as shall, by resolution of its board of Supervisors duly adopted, so provide." In other words, define the position of county nurse as optional, not mandatory. They wanted relief from the expenses of a county nurse, reasoning that "the taxes in the rural communities in the northern part of Wisconsin are now so burdensome that the people are almost unable to bear the same."[41] The petitions from local women's groups, Gardner's open letter, and her appearance before the county board resulted in the restoration of her salary in 1923.

Unfortunately, by the next year, the legislative situation had changed dramatically. Many Wisconsin counties in the 1920s found themselves strapped financially. They, including Price County, again petitioned the state legislature to make the position of county nurse voluntary. The state complied, and when the mandatory aspect of the law was dropped in 1924, many counties discontinued the service. In describing the situation in Price County, the state nurse reported:

> In May 1924, the county board abolished the office to take effect at the expiration of the nurse's contract [31 August 1924]. No criticism was expressed regard[ing] the nurse, or her work. It was presented as a matter of economy. Many of the new members of the board has [sic] been elected on an economy platform.[42]

County supervisors were not questioning the benefits of having a county nurse; they did not claim that the position was a waste of money, merely that it cost money. In a sense, Gardner's tax-paying arguments in 1923 supported the board's decision in 1924. If Gardner had argued the case differently in 1923, if she had emphasized its value to the county's health and welfare rather than its tax advantages, would the county board have not abolished the office in 1924? That is unlikely. The counties in northern Wisconsin in particular were financially stressed. The state nurse's report explained that "With so much poverty, the continuous clamour [sic] for tax reduction offers every activity which will make a showing to their [the Supervisors'] constituents." She continued that "a mile of cement roads less would provide the funds for county nursing service for over five years, but this is less spectacular and to [sic] they are dependent on roads."[43] It was not that the county leaders did not understand the need for a county nurse, it was not that the residents did not appreciate all her services, but eliminating the office was merely an easy way to reduce the county budget.

This major setback did not deter Gardner from her work. She did not slow her pace and even added to it. In 1924 she arranged the 3-week visit to Price County of the State Health Department's Child Welfare Special. The highly popular Child Welfare Special brought state doctors and nurses to rural areas for several days or weeks. Again, this was public health, not intended to interfere with the medical practice of local physicians. Thus, doctors and nurses would examine children and instruct mothers on appropriate childcare and direct them to area doctors, if warranted, for further diagnosis or treatment. Morgan had scheduled the Special to work in Price County from August 25 to September 12. However, visits were predicated on the presence of a county nurse "because the work of the Child Welfare Special is far more effective if there is a county nurse to do the follow-up work," Morgan reminded Gardner shortly before the board's vote. There were many counties with nurses still on the waiting list, and the Special could accomplish much in those counties.[44] Given the May vote to abolish the position, it appeared that the Child Welfare Special would not come to Price County. And yet, it did come, though the dates were moved up so that all the weeks were in August, when Gardner was there. With her commitment to the county and to public health education, it is quite likely that Gardner impressed upon the state officials the importance of the Special's visit for Price County and convinced the State Board of Health that the trailer would be useful, even without a county nurse to do follow-up.

The detailed preparations for a visit from the Special added significantly to Gardner's other duties, preparations she took on willingly.[45] She placed notices in the local newspapers, announcing the dates of the visit and telling women where they could make appointments. She identified local women to assist in organizing appointments, to canvas the neighborhood for others who might need appointments, and then to transport the families, if necessary, to the site of the Special on the day of their appointments. She located interpreters who would be available in communities with non-English-speaking clients.[46] She also arranged each site in advance.

Gardner found that all the work was well worth the efforts. She proudly proclaimed:

> The mothers of Price County have waited two years for the coming of the State Board of Health Child Welfare Special. That interest has not waned has been shown by the good attendance the first week, despite the poor weather . . . 174 children were examined the first week.[47]

In her notes to the local women who assisted her with the Special, she expressed her gratitude for their service and her recognition that "the mothers fully appreciated the coming of the Special." Unfortunately,

> The records [of each examination] will be left in the office. I regret that there is no one to do the follow-up work, as some of the cases should be under observation for sometime [sic] to derive benefit from the coming of the Special.[48]

Despite her disappointment, Gardner gleefully wrote about the "very pleasant and profitable three weeks" she spent with the Special and its staff. "I am so glad," she continued, "that the Special could come while I was still in Price County, and that we could have as busy as last three weeks as we have had."[49] On September 1, 1924, Price County lost a county nurse, but public health nursing did not lose Gardner; she immediately moved into the position of County Nurse of Forest County.

CONCLUSION

From 1919 to 1924, Ernestine Kandel and Teresa Gardner provided Price County with an ever-expanding array of public health and social welfare services. From all reports these nurses established the position of county nurse as an integral part of the community structure. Clients, health practitioners, teachers, judges, and neighbors recognized that the nurses were critical to the health and welfare of the county. True, the county was financially strapped, undoubtedly a critical factor in the demise of the position. Yet other adjacent counties were also hard pressed to raise the necessary tax revenues and they were able to maintain a county nurse. Forest County, for instance, is also in the northern reaches of Wisconsin. The State Department of Health's 1927 analysis of the condition in Price County points to another nonfinancial factor: no focal point of support, or, as the report described it, "An active representative organization principally interested in health promotion might insure [sic] this important service to the county."[50]

The histories of Kandel and Gardner document that many in the county recognized health needs and many called upon the nurses to satisfy those needs. With so many attempting to direct it, the office of county nurse lacked a clear definition and, thus, it was relatively easy for interested parties to make more demands and extend the job further. Upon leaving Price County, Gardner remarked that she had enjoyed the work "but the field is so large and so much you wish to accomplish is left undone for lack of funds and time, that at times the work is depressing."[51] It was difficult for a single person, even a highly competent person, to sustain a job "so large," with "so much . . . to accomplish," and at the same time ill-defined and so easily expanded. A focused infrastructure was needed to support the position and its necessary boundaries. The public health framework did not arrive in Price County until the late 1930s, when the position of county nurse was reintroduce.

NOTES

1. Letter from Teresa Gardner to Dr. J. T. Speck, dated November 29, 1922, located in the Wisconsin Historical Society Archives, Price County (Wisconsin), Dept. of Public Welfare, County Nurse case files, 1920–1924, Series 25 (hereafter referred to as Price Series 25), box 3, folder 27.

2. Laws of Wisconsin, 1913, chap. 93.

3. Laws of Wisconsin, 1919, chap. 311.

4. Another early county to appoint a county nurse was Lincoln County, which appointed Theta Mead in 1917. However, Mead was an unusual appointment in that she had been a resident of that county and in private practice there for several years before her appointment. Most of the women who became Wisconsin county nurses moved into the locale upon their appointments, often making them outsiders to local officials and residents. For Mead's biography, see Joan Jensen, "The World of Theta Mead, County Nurse," *Wisconsin Magazine of History* 92, no. 3 (Spring 2009): 2–15.

5. Letter from Teresa Gardner to Mary P. Morgan, Director of the Wisconsin Child Welfare Bureau, dated June 21, 1924, Price Series 25, box 1, folder 24.

6. The description of Kandel's first month is drawn from "Ernestine Kandel, Price County Nurse, Phillips, Wisconsin, August [1919] Report," located in the Wisconsin Historical Society Archives, Price County (Wisconsin), Dept. of Public Welfare, County Nurse's monthly reports, 1919–1924, 1947–1949, Price Small Series 12 (hereafter referred to as Price Series 12), folder 1.

7. Public health nurses in this period were particularly cautious to differentiate their work—preventive medicine and health instruction—from that of the physician, that is, diagnostic and therapeutic.

8. *The Modern Health Crusade: A National Program of Health Instruction in Schools*, 5th ed. (New York, NY: National Tuberculosis Association, 1922). This manual appears to be basically similar to earlier editions.

9. Kandel is quoted in "Scrubbing Ears Now Popular," *Park Falls Independent*, 20 January 1921.

10. Ernestine Kandel, Price County Nurse, Phillips, Wisconsin, August [1919] Report, Price Series 12, folder 1.

11. Kandel, Price County Nurse, August [1919].

12. Kandel, Price County Nurse, August [1919].

13. Ernestine Kandel, Price County Nurse, Phillips, Wisconsin, January [1920] Report, Price Series, 12, folder 1.

14. Kandel, Price County Nurse, January [1920].

15. Letter Gardner to Morgan, dated June 23, 1922, Price Series 25, box 1, folder 24.

16. Rima D. Apple, *Perfect Motherhood: Science and Childrearing in America* (New Brunswick, NJ: Rutgers University Press, 2006).

17. Letter from Gardner to Morgan, Director, dated June 21, 1924, Price Series 25, box 1, folder 24. The classes probably used Mary P. Morgan, *Outline of Course on Infant Care for Use in Little Mothers' Classes* (Madison, WI: Wisconsin State Board of Health, 1920).

18. Letter from W. J. M. to "County Nurse," dated June 12, 1923, Price Series 25, box 3, folder 2.

19. Nurse's narrative report, initially dated June 14, 1923, Price Series 25, box 3, folder 2.

20. Nervine is a patent medicine developed in the 1880s by Franklin Miles, the founder of the pharmaceutical company Miles Laboratories. It was marketed as late as the 1960s as a "calmative." A Google search on May 2, 2013, identified several products still marketed under this name, though not associated with Miles Laboratories or its successors.

21. Nurse's narrative report, June 14, 1923.

22. Nurse's narrative report, June 14, 1923.

23. Letter from H. R. to "County Nurse," dated June 18, 1923, Price Series 25, box 3, folder 2.

24. Nurse's narrative report, June 14, 1923.

25. Kandel, Price County Nurse, September [1919].

26. Kandel, Price County Nurse, February [1920].

27. Letter from Mrs. O. W. H. to Miss Kindall [sic], dated August 22, 1921, Price Series 25, box 1, folder 71.

28. Letter from Mrs. R. to Gardner, dated December 9, 1923, and Gardner's report dated December 11, 1923, both located in Price Series 25, box 3, folder 4.

29. Kandel, Price County Nurse, September [1919].

30. Letter from G. K. to Kandel, dated July 4, 1921, Price Series 25, box 2, folder 17.

31. Letter from Morgan to Teresa Gardner, dated April 10, 1922, Price Series 26, box 1, folder 24.

32. Memo from Morgan, "Subject: Standing Orders for Public Health Nurses," dated January 5, 1922, Price Series 25, box 2, folder 62.

33. Letter from F. W. Mitchell to Gardner, dated December 15, 1921, Price Series 25, box 2, folder 47.

34. Letter from Gardner to Speck, dated January 28, 1922, Price Series 25, box 3, folder 27.

35. "Second Nurse Is Needed in County," *Park Falls Independent*, August 12, 1920.

36. Letter from [Kandel] to Morgan, dated April 25, 1921, Price Series 26, box 1, folder 24.

37. "Resolution adjusting salary of County Nurse," No. 872, submitted by A. W. Resimius, text located in Wisconsin Historical Society Archives, Price County (Wisconsin), Clerk, Original proceedings and papers of the County Board, 1885–1959, Price Series 26 (hereafter referred to as Price Series 26), box 7, folder 10.

38. Petitions are located in Price Series 26, box 7, folder 11.

39. Petitions from Women's Christian Temperance Union and St. Margaret's Guild may be found in Price Series 26, box 7, folder 11.

40. Gardner, "Communication: Saving the Taxpayer," *The Phillips Times* 2 (June 1923). See also "County Nurse Gives Facts about Work," undated clipping located in Price Series 25, box 2, folder 78.

41. "Resolution No. 841," typescript located in Price Series 26, box 7, folder 6.

42. "Price County," typescript history [dated August 1927], located in the Wisconsin Historical Society Archives, Wisconsin. Public Health Nursing Section, District advisory nurses narrative reports, 1925–1968, Series 908 (hereafter referred to as Series 908), box 3, folder: Price County.

43. "Price County," typescript history [dated August 1927], Series 908, box 3, folder: Price County.

44. Letter from Morgan to Gardner, dated April 28, 1924, located in Price Series 25, box 1, folder 24.

45. A sample of letters documenting her work can be found in Price Series 25, box 1, folder 23.

46. In 1920, the population of Price County was 18,517, of which 25% were foreign-born.

47. Press release, dated August 21, 1924, located in Price Series 25, box 1, folder 41.

48. One example of this is the letter from Gardner to Miss Laina M. Pajunen, dated August 29, 1924, Price Series 25, box 1, folder 23.

49. Letter from Gardner to Morgan, dated August 29, 1924, located in Price Series 25, box 1, folder 23.

50. "Price County," typescript history [dated August 1927], Series 908, box 3, folder: Price County.

51. Letter from Gardner to Morgan, dated June 11, 1924, located in Price Series 25, box 1, folder 24.

3

· · · · ·

School Nursing in Virginia:
Hookworm, Tooth Decay, and
Tonsillectomies

· · · · ·

MARY E. GIBSON

Their practical suggestion was that a nurse should work with the physician, carrying out under his orders the treatment for simple cases, without excluding them from school, and following to their homes the more serious cases of eye, head, or skin trouble, seeing that they received medical attention, teaching the mother, when this should be necessary, and keeping a record of the time the child was absent, not allowing it to remain out of school longer than necessary.[1]

IN 1902 NURSE LEADER LAVINIA DOCK described the "school nurse experiment" in the *American Journal of Nursing*. The experiment was an attempt to meet the needs of children in urban industrialized areas where poverty and overcrowding, as well as the rise of factories and child labor, created a setting in which children were not always valued and their health needs were often ignored. Children suffered from a variety of conditions ranging from pediculosis, impetigo, ringworm, eczema, and diseases of the eye. Discharging ears and wounds, defective vision and hearing, orthopedic defects, and contagious diseases such as measles and tuberculosis all threatened the children's ability to learn. To help alleviate this burden of disease, many urban schools initiated physical inspection of children on a regular basis.[2]

ORIGINS OF SCHOOL NURSING

In the early 20th century, Lillian Wald, founder of New York's Henry Street Settlement, recognized the challenge physicians faced in treating the health needs of the city's school children. Through their inspections, physicians identified large numbers of children with health problems. When they identified problems the medical inspectors' only strategy was to exclude the child from school and provide a card for the child to take home. These cards merely stated the diagnosis and the recommendation that parents take their child for treatment. Many parents who were not literate or fluent in English did not understand the significance of the message and often ignored or put aside the cards. As a result, there was absolutely no assurance that the child's condition would be addressed by a professional or that the child would be isolated if the disease was contagious.[3] Excluded children also missed classes, often for extended periods of time.

From her experience with the Henry Street Settlement, Wald understood the issues surrounding the lack of health care for school children and its significance regarding the overall health of the community. At the same

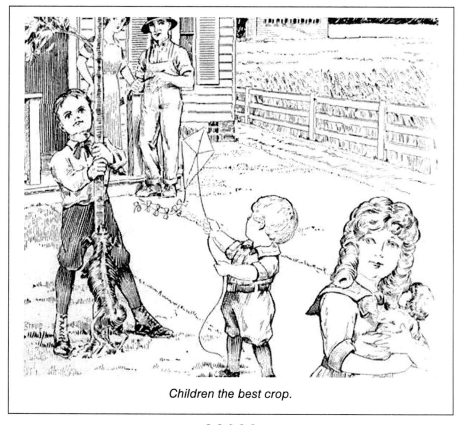

Children the best crop.

• • • • •

time, she also recognized the potential role nurses could play in addressing the school children's health. Rather than have the children excluded from school waiting "on the doorsteps to play with their classmates," or "romping with them through the halls of the tenement" when well-meaning but over-worked mothers could not supervise them, Wald proposed that nurses see children in schools and follow up with them through home visits.[4]

In October 1902, Wald sent Henry Street nurse Lina Rogers into four neighborhood schools in a 1-month demonstration project. The school nurse experiment substantially reduced the number of children excluded from school. Within weeks, a corps of 11 nurses, sponsored by the Board of Health and assisted by the Board of Education, began work in the New York City schools.[5] Within 1 year, the number of children excluded from school for health reasons decreased by 90%, thus establishing school nursing as the "link needed to complete the chain of medical inspection."[6] The project met both the goals of educators to keep children in school, as well as the goals of public health officials to improve child health. By 1909, 141 nurses worked in the 458 schools of New York City, cooperating with the school principals and medical inspectors.[7]

RURAL SCHOOLS

Conventional beliefs held that rural children, with access to fresh air, clean water, and farm-fresh food, were healthier than urban children.[8] However, historical evidence documents that rural children suffered greater morbidity and mortality than their city counterparts.[9] Hookworm, pellagra, and malaria were endemic in many southern states, while smallpox and tuberculosis, among other communicable diseases, were also prevalent.[10] The residents of isolated rural areas frequently lacked access to a physician, hospital, or nurse. Moreover, in the early 20th century, few rural families had sanitary privies or clean drinking water.

The problems found in homes carried over to the schools. Rural schools were often located in isolated areas and not subject to inspection or modern building codes. The one-room schools often lacked proper lighting, heat, and ventilation. Many times the classrooms did not even have desks. Children in these rural schools had limited or no access to medical or nursing care, and uncorrected conditions, such as skeletal deformities, infected tonsils, and vision defects, hindered their ability to learn.

ADVANCES IN SCHOOL HEALTH

The advancement of health and education occurred in tandem in the Commonwealth of Virginia. In 1902, like many southern states, Virginia adopted a new constitution that advanced a more progressive agenda related to schools and health in the state.[11] Assertive, often wealthy urban women also played a significant role in pushing for educational and health reform, as did northern philanthropists. During his governorship, former school teacher Claude Swanson (1906–1910) made significant reforms in education and health, including the reorganization of the State Department of Health.[12]

In Virginia, school nursing began in the city of Richmond in 1909 when the Instructive Visiting Nurses Association (IVNA) employed Ann Gulley, RN. She worked in two Richmond schools examining 750 students and referring 291 to specialists. As a result of the changes Gulley made to improve the attendance and health of the students, the IVNA soon loaned two nurses to the Richmond schools. The city health department later assumed responsibility for the schools and provided nursing coverage.[13] The idea of school nursing spread to other areas including Loudon County in northern Virginia, which would become a pioneer in county school nursing. There, a group of concerned citizens in the Quaker church first sponsored the school nurse experiment employing Mrs. McCulley, RN. Later the county school board shared the cost of the nurse.[14] Clearly, school nursing continually relied upon a combination of private and public funding.

HOOKWORM AND SANITARY SURVEYS

Between 1909 and 1914 the Commission for the Eradication of Hookworm, sponsored by the Rockefeller Sanitary Commission (RSC) and in cooperation with the State Health Department, worked to address hookworm infestation in Virginia's children. Hookworm, endemic in the South, led to childhood anemia and weight loss, sapping the infected children's energy and reducing their efficiency and ability to learn. Hookworm was transmitted through soil contaminated by infected feces, which carried the eggs of the hookworm. Once hatched, these larvae entered the body through the soft tissue between the toes, or by direct ingestion. Frequently barefoot and lacking sanitary provisions (e.g., sanitary privies), rural Virginians perpetuated hookworm infection.

The Commission's surveys showed that of more than a half million children examined in the South, 39% were infected.[15] Entire families carried the infection. Examinations in Orange County, Virginia, in 1913 indicated that approximately 24% of the boys were infected with hookworm and about 20% of the girls; when divided between Black and White children, infection rates indicated that 25% of Whites and 19% of Blacks were infected.[16] One *Virginia Health Bulletin*, a circular provided to Virginia homes to enlighten the population concerning public health issues, stated, "Perhaps the greatest enemy of efficiency in our rural schools today is hookworm disease."[17]

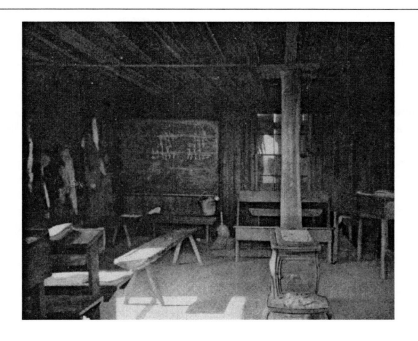

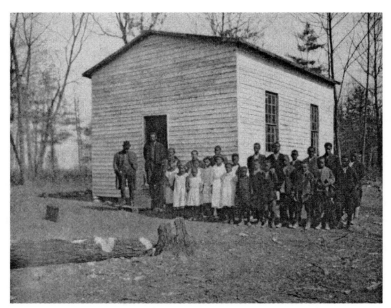

A typical school in Orange County.
Source: Sanitary Survey of the Schools of Orange County, VA, United States Bureau of Education Bulletin, 1914.

● ● ● ● ●

The hookworm campaign also addressed broader issues of child health in the Commonwealth. Through the school inspections for hookworm, other health issues such as poor vision, dental deficiencies, and malnutrition were identified. In 1914, the Annual Report of the Health Commissioner to the Governor of Virginia acknowledged that the work had not eliminated hookworm, but "at the very least we have reached that state of popular education where a very earnest interest in hookworm disease . . . is the best possible guarantee that the States will build on the foundation which the Rockefeller Sanitary Commission has laid."[18] While the Sanitary Commission's campaign was not successful in eradicating hookworm, it did lead to public health education and provisions for improved sanitation in the countryside, and ultimately led to the formation of health units, providing access to care for Virginians living in remote areas of the state. After the commission completed its work in 1914, Rockefeller money from the International Health Board supported rural public health. Hookworm and other physical conditions continued to be monitored, often by school nurses. As a result, not only was hookworm prevalence reduced, but other health measures became standard in rural schools.

In the same year, the *U.S. Bureau of Education Bulletin* published a report on a "Sanitary Survey of the Schools of Orange County, Virginia,"[19] authored by Roy Flannagan, MD, Director of Inspections.[20] The report documented that the schools in Orange County demonstrated an average sample of Virginia schools. It also noted that the 42 schools inspected were in abysmal physical condition. Only 2,600 of the county's 4,000 school-age children were enrolled, and during the 1913 inspections only 1,800 were in attendance, reflecting a 30% to 40% absentee rate.

The report further documented that most school sessions were between 5 and 6 months long. Poor ventilation and inadequate lighting and furnishings were the norms for the primarily one-room school houses. Wood stoves heated all the schools. Eighteen schools had unsanitary privies, and six schools had no privy of any kind. In addition, the water supplies of all the schools were insufficiently protected from surface pollution.[21] Flannagan wrote collectively of the county schools, "For the most part these schools are located in the midst of woods or on bleak, windswept hillsides, remote from dwellings . . . in . . . splendid isolation."[22] Their locations, in places called Raccoon Ford, Burr Hill, Indian Town, Old Mine Run, and Wilderness, bespoke their remoteness.

The study of the Orange County schools also involved the children's physical condition. Each school averaged only about 15 students. The examinations revealed that 25% of White children and 38% of Black children were malnourished, and of all children, 17.5% were anemic.[23] Additional physical deficiencies included nose and throat problems (31%–35%), tooth decay (42%–58%), eye defects, including vision or more serious problems (26%), and lung disease (37%). Sixty-eight percent of the children had been vaccinated for smallpox.

Despite the efforts of the Rockefeller Foundation's hookworm campaign, hookworm continued to plague the South for the next several decades. Reporting on her work with the county public health officer, the sanitary inspector of the county, and the superintendent of schools, one nurse in Pittsylvania County, Virginia, reported on her work:

> Loaded with two suitcases and portable scales, we drive up to a school house. The building is unpainted and rather dilapidated looking. . . . After making a mental survey of pupils, we can usually give a good guess as to the infections to be found . . . and endeavor to get a specimen of each child's bowel movement. . . . They [specimens] are examined, and should an infection be found, a notice is sent to the parents. . . . If the treatment is indicated, we send it to him free, following the family up, examining, probably treating and curing them. Occasionally, we find children . . . whose parents cannot read or write. These families we follow and endeavor to explain to them the importance of examination for hookworm.[24]

The nurse noted that of the 16% of those infected, approximately 40% accepted the free treatment.

In 1916 Jane Ranson, RN, became the first director of the Bureau of Public Health Nursing for Virginia. Her first strategy included visiting localities in the state where public health nursing was in place and recording the progress of the nurses. She enlisted the cooperation of public health nurses, asking them to send regular reports of their work so she could follow the overall progress of public health nursing in Virginia.[25] These voluntary reports showed that the locales and sites of public health care were funded by numerous sources, including private philanthropy; socially conscious religious groups; mothers' clubs; civic groups; and a few by public dollars.

During her visits, Ranson determined that public health nurses throughout the state practiced in four specialty areas: school nursing, visiting nursing, specialty nursing (including tuberculosis and baby care), and industrial nursing. She also found that 88 public health nurses practiced in Virginia. Ranson wrote that school nursing provided the "biggest returns for the money,"[26] particularly in rural areas. She advocated for public funds to support these nurses. However, throughout the Commonwealth school nurses received support from various public and private sources well into the 1920s.[27]

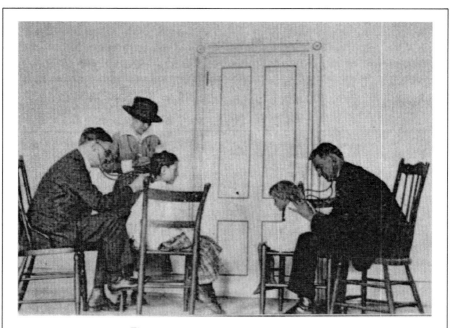

The examination of school children.
Source: Annual Report of the State Board of Health and the State Health Commissioner to Governor of Virginia, 1920.

● ● ● ● ●

Physical assessment soon became a key aspect of the nurses' work. By the 1920s, nurses and teachers recorded children's weight, height, and physical conditions. The 1918 West Law had mandated that by 1925 *teachers* would perform rudimentary physical assessments on students with the referral and follow-up assigned to nurses.[28] Some counties instituted the "five point" child program, documenting five measures: healthy vision, hearing, weight, teeth, and tonsils and adenoids. For example, in the first 6 months of 1920, Albemarle County school nurse Lily Jones inspected the students in 28 schools for these and additional markers, and found defects of teeth, eyesight, tonsils, pale skin color, nasal obstruction, malnutrition, infectious diseases, and ear problems. Jones also assisted the physician in the inspection of the remaining school children of the county.[29] Nurses provided the follow-up for these inspections, impressing parents of the need for corrections.

TRANSPORTATION AND DISTANCES

Challenges included the vast distances and poor roads the nurses were required to travel in order to reach remote communities. One estimate described travel as consuming one third of the nurses' time.[30] By necessity, the number of visits to some schools or homes was limited because of their remote locations. While village schools could be visited as often as once a month, some one-room rural schools could be visited only two to three times a year. In some cases, the nurses had to ride on horseback to reach isolated schools or families. Blanche Webb, a Red Cross supervising nurse visiting Bath County, Virginia, in February described how Star Chapel could only be reached on horseback: "I [was] full of wonder and admiration for the nurse who, each day, in bad weather and good, takes the trail and finds the people; for truly it is not easy to reach schools through the mountains, on roads impassable by automobile or buggy. . . . "[31] Indeed, long distances and the "chronic poor condition" of the roads were factors that ultimately inhibited the progress of rural nursing, not only in Virginia, but also in many regions of the country.[32]

Part of the follow-up included transporting children great distances to access medical clinics and hospitals. In 1923 Lillian Gorton, RN, of Caroline County reported that she made a 170-mile round trip to Richmond with several children who needed medical treatment. She transported a little girl with crossed eyes, an 11-year-old boy who was nearly blind, a child requiring a checkup for his eyes after receiving glasses, and a mother and her infant who needed surgery for a cleft palate. After delivering the mother and baby to hospital admissions, she accompanied the other children to their various appointments.

The distances and the rough terrain provided significant challenges. During the trip the car had a broken spring and a leaking radiator in addition to two separate blow outs requiring replacement. Having begun her day at 7:00 a.m., Gorton finally completed the trip at 10:30 in the evening when she returned the last child home.[33] Rural nursing was not for the faint of heart.

SPECIALTY CLINICS

School nurses also ensured that children received specialized care, sometimes in clinics funded or partially funded by the state health department.[34] The nurses arranged vaccination and dental clinics, as well as clinics to address problems of tonsils and adenoids. As examples, in Fauquier County, school nurse Agnes Kloman organized dental clinics,[35] and in Accomac County in 1923, 27 children underwent tonsillectomies/adenoidectomies in a high school building's auditorium, specially fitted as an operating room for the day. A specialist from Maryland performed the operations assisted by eight local doctors. Two neighboring county nurses helped Sara Crosley, RN, and local volunteers care for the children before and after surgery.[36]

GAINING ACCESS TO FAMILIES

School nursing actually provided nurses with the means to identify families with health care needs. As public health officials in Virginia noted, "A nurse with this experience can go into the home without being regarded as an intruder and can do a work utterly beyond the reach of the medical inspector."[37] The school child was not the only focus of the work and "good family health work" could be done at each visit.[38] Family health work required enlisting the cooperation of the mother; mothers who were isolated and alone were receptive to the nurses' visits.[39] School nurses in remote rural areas were often called upon to manage all health care needs in a community. For these nurses, the organizational and professional challenges required them to work to the full extent of their training.[40]

Health Commissioner Ennion Williams, MD, described the extent of the Virginia school nurse's role,

> First is the school nurse, whose primary duty is to visit the schools of the county or city, to examine the children for the more obvious physical defects and to urge upon parents the correction for these defects before they become seated. In a larger sense, the school nurse is a sanitary educator, occupying a strategic position and opening the way for more adequate organization. It is our belief that the school is the first place for the nurse to begin her work. We have reached this conclusion because . . . by operating in the schools she can reach a considerable element of the population in a very short while. More than this, the school offers, perhaps, the most effective point of contact between sanitation and the home. The nurse who comes to plead for the treatment of a child is accorded a welcome which a regular health inspector or a health officer cannot hope to receive. Furthermore, the school nurse can do her chief work among those who will show the greatest benefits from adequate preventive measures, and at the same time have open minds wherewith to receive the great and salutary lessons of modern sanitation.[41]

In 1916, Williams declared the public health nurses in the state "missionaries of public health" and "an indispensable cog in the machinery for the prevention and cure of disease" in the communities where they practiced.[42] In the process of their duties, the nurses identified families in need and referred them to local charities. As public health nurses, they assessed the whole family, through social, health, and economic lenses.

Experts and nurses agreed that the role of the rural nurse required the best educated and most experienced nurses, and that the school nurse was the most effective way to introduce public health nursing in a rural setting.[43]

In 1917, one rural nurse stated, "In a great many cases, the children are the only means of reaching the homes, sometimes situated in such out of the way places that it is hard to find them."[44] Through her work, the isolated rural family could be introduced to the gospel of health and sanitation. According to Mary Gardner, a public health nurse who wrote extensively about public health nursing and its relationship to the health of the family, "The school has been found . . . the best door of entry. School work has the advantage of giving the quickest introduction and producing the most tangible results. . . . "[45] Furthermore, nurses were well received by parents.

FINANCIAL BARRIERS

Financial barriers also challenged the school health programs and the nurses' work. Local financial prosperity or a supportive public often determined if there would be funding for school nurses. In many instances, there was no local infrastructure to assist in funding a health department. Payment for the services of school nurses often depended upon the local boards of education, local civic and/or religious organizations, mothers' clubs, parent–teacher associations, the local Red Cross, or a combination of these sources of funding. Many counties relied on piecemeal and temporary financial resources to support school health programs, while still other counties were never able to find the necessary resources.

CONCLUSION

Virginia, stretching from isolated mountain villages and hollows on the west, to the coastal eastern shores, and from the tobacco fields of the south, to the oyster beds of the Chesapeake Bay, presented its own challenges to providing access to care for its rural citizens.

Local efforts to improve sanitation, cure parasitic infections, and promote clean water were enhanced by national programs and by philanthropy, and became more effective as state health departments became better organized. Transportation and remote locations limited the ability of patients to reach medical and nursing clinics and for nurses to reach patients. Furthermore, environmental conditions often caused or perpetuated poor health, both in schools and in rural homes. School nursing provided an opportunity for nurses to identify children's health needs. It also gave nurses an entree into communities through their home visits. The frequent hesitation of parents to permit modern treatment and limited available funding did not stop rural nurses, even if it meant transporting families over long distances.

As public health nursing became more standardized, and as state funds and supplemental philanthropy allowed, county health departments developed and provided more nurses who could promote child health and provide access to care throughout the Commonwealth.

NOTES

1. Lavinia Dock, "School Nurse Experiment in New York," *American Journal of Nursing* 3, no. 2 (1902): 109.

2. S. W. Newmayer, "The Trained Nurse in the Public Schools as a Factor in the Education of the Children," *American Journal of Nursing* 7, no. 3 (December 1906): 185–91.

3. Lina Rogers, "Some Phases of School Nursing," *American Journal of Nursing* 8, no. 12 (September 1909): 966–74.

4. Lillian Wald, "Medical Inspection of Public Schools," *Annals of the American Academy of Political and Social Sciences* 25 (March 1905): 91.

5. Lina Rogers, "School Nursing in New York City," *American Journal of Nursing* 3, no. 6 (March 1903): 448–50.

6. Rogers, "Phases of School Nursing," 966; Rogers, "School Nursing in New York City," 448–50.

7. Anna Kerr, "School Nursing in New York City," *American Journal of Nursing* 10, no. 2 (November 1909): 106–8.

8. Ch. Wardell Stiles, "The Rural Health Movement," *Annals of the American Academy of Political and Social Science* 37, no. 2 (1911): 123–26; Taliaferro Clark, "The Physical Care of Rural School Children," *Public Health Reports* 38, no. 22 (June 1, 1923): 1181–190.

9. Elizabeth Cannon, "The Field of Rural Nursing," *The Public Health Nurse* 13, no. 3 (March 1921): 129–34.

10. Clark, "The Physical Care of Rural School Children," 1181.

11. Raymond Pulley, *Old Virginia Restored: An Interpretation of the Progressive Impulse 1870–1930* (Charlottesville, VA: University of Virginia Press, 1968), 66–8.

12. William Link, *A Hard Country and a Lonely Place* (Chapel Hill, NC: UNC Press, 1986), 96. Reorganization of the State Health Department occurred in 1908.

13. Tompkins McCaw Library Historical Collections, Virginia Commonwealth University, Richmond, VA, IVNA Collection, Box 8, Folder 3.

14. *Report of State Commissioner of Health to the Governor of Virginia* (1916) (Richmond, VA, 1917), 135.

15. C. Vann Woodward, *Origins of the New South* (Baton Rouge, LA: LSU Press, 2000), 427.

16. Roy Flannagan, "Sanitary Survey of the Schools of Orange County, VA," *US Bureau of Education Bulletin* 17, whole no. 590 (Washington, DC: Government Printing office, 1914), 26–7.

17. "The Sanitary School," *Virginia Health Bulletin* VI, no. 10 (October 1914): 181.

18. *Annual Report of the Health Commissioner of Virginia to the Governor*, chap. II (Richmond, VA, 1914).

19. Flannagan, "Sanitary Survey of the Schools of Orange County," 26–7.

20. Flannagan, "Sanitary Survey of the Schools of Orange County," 7. Flannagan was accompanied in his inspection work by two Rockefeller Sanitary Commission doctors, the superintendent of Orange schools and three faculty physicians from the University of Virginia, along with a dentist from the county. No nurses are noted in the report. It is important to note here that there was not a Bureau of Public Health Nursing yet established at the Virginia State Health Department, so any nurse practicing in Orange or other counties did not have a central reporting strategy or a coordinating body.

21. Flannagan, "Sanitary Survey of the Schools of Orange County," 23.

22. Flannagan, "Sanitary Survey of the Schools of Orange County," 22.

23. Flannagan, "Sanitary Survey of the Schools of Orange County," 26–7.

24. Kate Hall, "Saving the Child from Hookworm," *The Public Health Nurse* 12, no. 11 (1920): 951–53.

25. Nurses were supported by local funds, private, secular, and church organizations, school boards, the Red Cross, Mother's leagues, and industry. *Report of the Health Commissioner to the Governor of Virginia* (Richmond, VA, 1916).

26. *Annual Report of the Health Commissioner to the Governor* (Richmond, VA, 1917), 169.

27. *Annual Report of the Health Commissioner to the Governor*, 170.

28. "The Teacher and the State Board of Health," *Virginia Health Bulletin* XIII, no. 6 (June 1921): 1.

29. *Annual Report of the Health Commissioner to the Governor of Virginia* (Richmond, VA, 1920) Appendix II.

30. C. A. Greenleaf, "School Health Work in a Rural County," *Journal of Educational Sociology* 3, no. 1 (1929): 44–59.

31. Blanche Webb, "Roaming Through Virginia with the Public Health Nurse," *The Public Health Nurse* 12 (1920): 839.

32. Greenleaf, "School Health Work," 44–59.

33. "One Day's Work," *The Virginia Health Bulletin* XV, extra no. 10 (July–August 1923): 13.

34. "How to Get Dental Clinics," *Virginia Health Bulletin* XIV, extra no. 8 (May 1922): 8.

35. "A Plan for Ambulatory Dental Clinics," *The Public Health Nurse* 13, no. 2 (February 1921): 16.

36. "With the Nurses," *The Virginia Health Bulletin* XV, extra no. 10 (July–August 1923): 10–11.

37. *Report of the State Commissioner of Health to the Governor of Virginia* (Richmond, VA, 1916), 29.

38. Mary S. Gardner, *Public Health Nursing* (New York, NY: Macmillan, 1936), 215.

39. Margaret McMillan, "School Nursing in England," *American Journal of Nursing* 11, no. 6 (March 1911): 159–64.

40. Ethlyn Cockrell, "One Morning with a School Nurse," *American Journal of Nursing* 23, no. 1 (August 1923): 959.

41. *Report of the State Commissioner of Health to the Governor of Virginia* (Richmond, VA, 1916), 69.

42. *Report of the State Commissioner of Health to the Governor of Virginia*, 70.

43. Annie Brainard, *The Evolution of Public Health Nursing* (Philadelphia, PA: WB Saunders, 1922), chap. 18; J. B. Gwin, "Rural Social Work," *Journal of Social Forces* 3, no. 2 (1925): 280–83.

44. Sybil Koeller, "Rural District Nursing," *American Journal of Nursing* 17, no. 4 (January 1917): 317.

45. Mary S. Gardner, *Public Health Nursing*, 3rd ed. (New York, NY: Macmillan, 1936), 215.

4

•••••

Nursing in Schoolfield Mill Village: Cotton and Welfare

•••••

SARAH WHITE CRAIG

"The very first workers placed in the field were a force of visiting nurses, which has proven a very wise move,"[1] noted Hattie Hylton, Director of Welfare work for Riverside Cotton Mills in Schoolfield, Virginia, when reporting on the progress the mills' nurses had made. In her 1915 report Hylton went on to note that, "by virtue of their profession" the nurses could win the trust of mill workers by visiting them in their homes.[2] Her comments testify to the fact that professional nurses played a vital role in providing both geographic and cultural access to health care for the thousands of textile mill workers in the post-Reconstruction South.

DEVELOPMENT OF AN INDUSTRIAL NURSING SPECIALTY

Lillian Wald worked tirelessly to define, highlight, and promote the industrial nursing specialty. Like other urban nurses, Wald routinely encountered the harsh realities of industrial working conditions. By the early 1900s, the need for care of the working poor was obvious to visiting nursing services throughout large urban centers like New York City.[3] Access to care for the working class was limited by availability of doctors, money to pay, and limited time to seek a doctor's care due to long work hours. The establishment of public health nursing grew from such needs that arose during American industrialization.

In June 1909, Lillian Wald expanded the growing role of the visiting nurse into industry.[4] Wald forged a cooperative relationship with New York's Metropolitan Life Insurance Company's director of welfare, Lee Frankel, enabling Henry Street nurses to visit working-class policy holders in the city. The Henry Street nurses followed up with these families and provided care as well as health education.[5] After 3 months of decreased trends in insurance claims, Metropolitan Life extended coverage of a visiting nursing service throughout New York City and by 1911 for policy holders across the United States, including the South.[6]

In addition to the Metropolitan Life collaboration, Lillian Wald and colleagues established first aid rooms on the Lower East Side of New York City in order to provide local workers with health services.[7] Wald's community first aid rooms met the health demands of the working people that otherwise went unnoticed.[8] Nurses managed first aid rooms by physicians' standing orders, and this level of autonomy required critical thinking and expert knowledge.[9] Large companies across the nation modeled nursing departments after Wald's industrial first aid rooms.[10] As the northern industrialists looked to the South to establish more mills, they carried with them the basics of industrial nursing practice.

THE SOUTHERN COTTON TEXTILE INDUSTRY: 1880–1930

Once established, the southern cotton industry grew rapidly between 1880 and 1930. In the late 1800s, as northern textile owners strove to outfit their mills with the latest technology, they began to explore opportunities to move their industry's production to the South. In need of cheap labor sources and natural resources, the mill owners discovered Virginia's Piedmont region,[11] a region that possessed an abundance of natural resources, including fast-moving rivers, access to raw cotton, and cheap labor as many farmers were seeking work. In addition, railroad connections to the North provided easy delivery of finished goods, making the Piedmont Valley an ideal place to establish cotton mills.[12] The region's resources had a great impact on the industry's prosperity—from its beginning in 1882 to 1899, the Riverside Cotton Mills in southern Virginia boasted the manufacturing of 23,133 bales of raw cotton via 66,650 spindles[13] and 2,771 looms.[14]

Traditionally, the South's economy was mostly agrarian, made up of small farms, with some larger plantations that generated cash crops of tobacco and cotton.[15] The majority of the small farms only yielded enough crops to sustain individual families who bartered and shared with neighbors to meet their needs. Jacquelyn Hall notes a "community quality of life" was present among these small farms.[16] However, by the 1880s farmers found they were no longer able to provide for their families; community quality of life was not enough to live on. The lack of financial stability eventually led many families to migrate to larger towns and cities in search of work and a better way of life. They left behind their poverty but brought with them their sense of community.[17] In years to come, as they struggled to adjust to the culture of an industrial society, their sense of community sustained them.

CULTURE, WORK, AND HEALTH IN SOUTHERN TEXTILE MILL VILLAGES

Southern community leaders had an ulterior motive in encouraging industrialization. They believed that railroad development and investment opportunities would stabilize the region's economy, and industrialization would "create a large white laboring class as a safeguard against the political possibilities of the large Negro population."[18] To an extent their plan succeeded. At the turn of the 20th century, the majority of southern mill employees were poor, White, and employed as spinners and weavers.[19] African Americans were also employed in the mills, but generally the only job available to them was considered the dirtiest job of all, namely unloading heavy bales from the cargo trains and opening the bales of raw cotton. Thus, the social mores of the South dictated that employment be based on race and class. Strengthened by the enforcement of the Jim Crow laws, these values continued to impact the textile industry into the 20th century and would further marginalize African American laborers.[20]

Following the example of other industrialists, textile mill owners established, built, and owned villages for their employees and their families. The mill villages were not alike; the availability and the quality of necessities and additional services varied from village to village. Basic services included, but were not limited to, housing, stores, schools, churches, and health care. Since many southern textile mills were situated in rural areas and often inaccessible to larger towns and cities, the company villages ultimately became the center of life for mill workers and their families. By the early 1900s, 92% of textile families lived in southern company-owned mill villages.[21] Many were transplanted Appalachian families who held fast to their cultural beliefs, resulting in many mill villages becoming a mix of rural values and those of the new industrial age. This mixed culture of the past and the present later presented a challenge to nurses and social workers who attempted to aid families and provide for their social welfare.

In the early 1900s, mill owners paid little attention to the health and welfare of their employees and working conditions were often poorly regulated. However, due to several devastating industrial accidents, labor safety began to slowly take form. By 1919, the U.S. Bureau of Labor began establishing sanitary and safety regulations for all U.S. industries. In textile mills these regulations included some basics: an adequate number of bathrooms for workers, at least one stool for every three female workers, air filtration to control dust in workrooms, and first aid cabinets.[22] The new regulations required that mill owners place guards over moving machinery parts, install proper lighting in workrooms and stairwells, and provide fire escapes in all factories greater than three stories high.[23] In 1918 the Virginia General Assembly passed additional legislation, in the form of workmen's compensation laws, to further protect the workers of the Commonwealth. These laws ultimately placed the responsibility and cost of job-related injury on the employer. As labor regulations increased, mill owners established safety precautions within the mills and created welfare departments to improve housing and provide medical and nursing services. Day care, social work, entertainment, and recreation were among other services provided by the company welfare departments. To address the health care issues surrounding the mill workers, the welfare departments employed professional nurses to care for the workers and their families.[24]

ESTABLISHING TRUST

Not all company welfare assistance was received graciously and openly by families. Culture played a significant role in how some mill families initially accepted those individuals. They were the most likely candidates to go out into the community, meet new families, and assess their living conditions and needs.[25] Often nurses' social calls to mill families' homes merely helped gain the families' confidence. The nurses essentially became the gatekeepers to the companies' welfare services, establishing trusting relationships between service providers and the mill workers. Through these relationships nurses were able to encourage more workers to utilize the available health care and welfare services.

AN UNSAFE ENVIRONMENT

Despite newly established labor laws and improved working conditions, many health risks for the mill workers and their families continued to exist. Work in cotton mills was dangerous and filthy. Automation of each step in making cotton cloth, from cotton ginning to weaving, increased production as well as the risks of injury and death. Workers risked falling or being pulled into the moving parts of the machines, which could crush, burn, cut, or even scalp them. Weavers and spinners worked 12-hour shifts, 6 days a week and night shifts in mills with electric lights.[26] The workers' long shifts resulted in fatigue, which played a role in accidents.

The air in the mill workrooms was filled with cotton dust, which led to many workers developing chronic cough.[27] Compounding this problem was the humid air that was kept at a constant 90 degrees. The high humidity[28] in the mills' workrooms prevented yarn from breaking, which resulted in costly machine repairs. The heat generated by the mills combined with the humid air created an ideal place for bacteria growth, resulting in a variety of infectious diseases. Textile workers experienced high rates of tuberculosis, chronic bronchitis, and pneumonia.[29] Unknown to the workers at the time, this was the first phase of byssinosis, commonly known as brown lung disease. Many workers with brown lung developed symptoms they casually referred to as a touch of asthma. But their breathing worsened over time until their activity tolerance diminished and finally they were no longer able to work.[30]

Other health problems attributed to the textile industry included hearing loss and fatigue. Weavers reported hearing loss and episodes of fatigue and nervousness from the constant hammering of looms.[31] Infectious, parasitic, and insect-borne diseases such as smallpox, malaria, tuberculosis, and hookworm also threatened the overall health of village residents. In many cases, illiteracy and poverty only worsened the situation. Unlike some industrial towns in the country, poor sanitation habits in the southern mill villages generally did not pose a problem; however, some company welfare programs included education programs for village residents that focused on sanitation and healthy habits.[32]

A NEED FOR IMPROVED NUTRITION

Dietary ailments were also prevalent in many southern mill villages. Limited income; the lack of fresh meat, milk, and eggs; or the lack of time to cultivate gardens to supplement their diets resulted in many mill families subsisting on dried meats and breads. These diets lacked essential niacin and led to rampant pellagra.[33] Unfortunately, few mill owners took notice of serious health issues such as pellagra unless the resultant illness affected the labor supply and ultimately the productivity of the mills. By 1915 an estimated 100,000 cases of pellagra were reported in the South. That same year, epidemiologist Joseph Goldberger identified poor diet as the root cause of pellagra and began working with southern boards of health to establish health education campaigns and improve the nutrition of rural residents, including those who lived in mill villages. Goldberger, local public health officials, and mill owners established pellagra stations throughout the South to ensure that more nutritious foods, at reasonable prices, were available to the residents.[34]

FOCUS ON SAFETY

Although larger mills in the South did offer some health benefits to workers such as a visiting nurse service or a village physician, this was not the norm.[35] As regulation of industrial safety progressed throughout the early 20th century, textile mill owners were required to provide a staffed first aid room to care for employees injured or taken ill while on the job. The first aid rooms, often established in a separate building on the premises and referred to as the community house or welfare building, became the center of health and recreation in many mill villages.[36] The mill nurses were responsible for organizing and equipping the first aid rooms with the common supplies of gauze, muslin, splints, slings, tourniquets, stretchers, scales, as well as stomach and rectal tubes. In addition, the nurses prepared, and had ready at all times, an emergency bag to take with them to the scene of any mill accident. The bags contained various dressings, medications, and tourniquets needed to treat accident victims.[37] The mill nurses, like other nurses located in industrial settings, reported to every accident. If the doctor was unable to be present, the nurse had the responsibility of providing emergency care. Emergencies in the cotton mills were not uncommon and included crushed or amputated limbs, shock, eye injuries, burns, and fainting. In such emergencies, the mill nurses, after gaining an understanding of the cause of the accidents and assessing the victims, had the knowledge and experience necessary to make decisions regarding the severity of the injuries and what steps needed to be taken. It was often the nurses' responsibility to decide whether to transport victims immediately to a hospital or to wait for a physician to arrive, as well as to carefully record orders, treatments, and observations. Thus, the nurses' actions were vital to the welfare of seriously injured mill workers.[38]

PRACTICING TO THE FULL EXTENT OF THEIR EDUCATION

In 1917 Lillian Wald wrote, "The industrial nurse is . . . not free to work except under the direction of a physician or surgeon. Her services should not be confined to first aid . . . In fact, her main function should be to conserve the health and lives of the workers . . . her work should include . . . regular conference hours during the working day, regular inspection of sanitary conditions, special attention to diet, charge of the hospital, and regular group instruction in health and hygiene."[39] As was true of all industrial nurses, nurses' work in the mills required them to practice to the fullest extent of their training in nursing and public health. Indeed, the boundaries between nursing and medicine blurred as nurses, unlike the company physician, lived in the village and their services were available and protected with standing orders at all times of the day and night. This issue of industrial nursing stepping into the practice of medicine was echoed throughout mill villages in the South, where the nurse was an economical liaison between mill and physician. In order to avoid disputes, new industrial nurses were taught to seek out local physicians upon their arrival to the mill village and to establish a working relationship. Most physicians in rural areas of the South appreciated the services that industrial and public health nurses provided in the populated industrial areas.[40]

Although physicians provided them with standing orders, the mill nurses administered medications in the first aid room only during emergencies[41] to avoid being accused of practicing medicine. The mill physicians created lists of available medications in the first aid rooms, which included boric acid, essence of peppermint, Jamaica ginger, white wine vinegar, bicarbonate of soda, iodine, alcohol, mercury, benzene, and petroleum jelly. Some physicians required the availability of hypodermic needles to administer stimulants when accident victims were in shock.

When workers were sent home due to illness or injury, the nurses required that the workers have someone at home to care for them. Therefore, in addition to their first aid room responsibilities, mill nurses also provided follow-up care to workers and their families in the home setting. These home visits gave the nurses the opportunity to assist in providing the necessary bedside care, as well the opportunity to assess the families' living conditions. At the request of some mill superintendents, nurses were also asked to make home visits to absent workers to confirm that the workers were indeed ill.[42]

The nurses' knowledge and understanding of the technology also made them the most likely to investigate and record why and how mill accidents occurred and to address safety conditions and potential risks with mill superintendents.[43] Accident reporting remained only a section of the industrial nurses' work as it related to prevention and safety. Nurses familiarized themselves with their specific state requirements due to variations in workmen's compensation and industrial regulations and maintained accurate documentation of events for reporting to the state. Accurate recordkeeping by the nurses was essential and became especially so after the enactment of the Workers' Compensation law.[44] It was the nurses' responsibility to carefully record orders, treatments, and observations—documentation that became important during workmen's compensation claims. In addition to

	—	I. Butts	6 Twist.	Hysterical	Rest in bed, taken home. Brother had enlisted and left for Canada to-day.
12 to 1	12/24	F. Fay	90 Tool	Emery, cornea, L.	Sent to eye specialist, Left off goggles.
	12/24	E. Day	10 Test.	Under weight	83 lbs. Saw Dr. T. 12/21 Brought well planned lunch. Adv. as to habits.
	12/26	D. Wat	97 Stenog.	Var. veins	Bandaged. Surgeon adv. no op. Measure for stocking next visit 8 A. M.

	1/8	G. Kane	56 SP.	Deserted by husband, 2 ch., 1 & 4, at day nursery. Referred to 12 Main St. re mother's pension. Foreman will allow time, P M. Following home visits made. See cards.

This sample entry from a nurse's daybook illustrates the detailed recordkeeping required of nurses in textile mills.[45]

● ● ● ● ●

providing documentation for compensation of injury and death, the nurses' data allowed for the trending of accident data both to identify mill areas requiring improvement in safety and to monitor for successful change.

HEALTH PROMOTION AND DISEASE PREVENTION

The work of the nurses went beyond the mill clinics and first aid rooms. They were also responsible for disease prevention within the mill villages and focused on educating the village residents on cancer, mental illness, and the prevention of infectious diseases.[46] Mill town nurses created maternal and child welfare programs based on the needs of the communities' residents. Many of the female workers and women in the village were first-time mothers with no female family members available to coach them through their first pregnancy. The nurses provided the women with prenatal care that included advising first-time mothers on what to expect during their pregnancy and encouraging them to visit the company doctors well before their actual labor.[47]

The nurses established well-baby clinics and provided checkups both in the welfare building and in the families' homes. The well-baby clinics, which were referred to as "Babies' Afternoon," focused on healthy weights, feeding schedules, and proper infant care. One mill nurse wrote that one of the greatest pleasures in her work was the time she spent on one street in the mill village when all of the women attended a class for new mothers. Later that summer, as she walked down the street, she noticed 10 babies in boxes and playpens in yards and on front porches. The nurse was thrilled that the new mothers had retained the information about the benefits of clean air and activity for babies and that none of the babies on the street had been sick once all summer.[48]

The nurses also visited mill schools and day care programs, examining the children. If needed, the nurses made appropriate referrals to local and regional physicians for further care. Infectious diseases, hookworm, and orthopedic and ear, nose, and throat referrals were the most common. Beyond attending to the immediate health care needs of the towns' citizens, the nurses also taught home nursing courses and sewing and cooking classes, thus addressing families' health through adequate clothing and nutrition.[49]

In an *American Journal of Nursing* article from 1930, a mill nurse described the work of nurses in mill towns to illustrate mill nurses' responsibilities. She used the case of a mill worker who came to the clinic for a minor finger laceration. After receiving the nurse's skillful care and appreciating her empathetic ear, the worker confided to the nurse that his wife was very ill with a lump on her neck, a jumping heart, nervousness, and frailty. He explained that she was seeing a "specialist" who charged her $10 a visit and she received powders that only lasted a short time, after which she would have to return and pay again. After repeated visits to the "specialist," the wife's condition had not improved, making the husband terribly frustrated. The next day, the nurse visited the wife at home and called on the specialist. She discovered that the specialist was not what he claimed to be and proceeded to refer the mill worker's wife to a regional hospital. There the surgeons removed the lump from her neck and prescribed medically appropriate treatment. The husband gave credibility to the nurse's practice as he began to tell his friends and coworkers how the mill nurse could also help their families.[50]

In general, White nurses attended to the needs of the poor, White mill workers, and their families. There is no evidence to suggest that nurses extended health services to Black workers. Most likely, the few Black workers at Dan River Mills in the early years obtained care from local Black doctors and nurses through the local Colored Charity and Welfare League.[51] As historian Patricia D'Antonio explained in a case study of Georgia nurses, southern women working as nurses for pay already went against the grain of southern social norms. It was socially not accepted for White women to care for Blacks during this time period in the South.[52]

SCHOOLFIELD VILLAGE, DAN RIVER MILLS, VIRGINIA

The leading cotton manufacturer in Virginia at the turn of the 20th century was Dan River Cotton Mills in Danville, Virginia.[53] In 1903 the mills' owners established the Schoolfield mill village to support the mills' immense growth. Schoolfield Village, named after President Robert Addison Schoolfield of the Danville Textile Mills, was often referred to as the model mill village. Its services expanded beyond basic living necessities and included a day nursery, a kindergarten, and a small hospital, exemplifying the company's early welfare program. Schoolfield provides an excellent case study to illustrate how successful such industrial welfare programs of the era could be. Located in the South's Piedmont region, Schoolfield became known as a flagship of southern industrial welfare.[54] In order to protect the mills' workforce and ultimately preserve the productivity of the mills, the mills' owners provided their employees welfare services, including health care.[55] Like other industrialists of the era, the mills owners' rationale for welfare benefits ranged from religious philanthropy to good business sense.[56]

In 1908 the mill owners appointed Hattie Hylton as superintendent of welfare work, and she immediately hired trained nurses to work with her in the welfare department.[57] The focus on nursing care was a new approach in the South. In many instances, early southern industries hired only a social worker who made social and sick calls, relying on local physicians and families to provide care for ill workers. Hylton identified the extensive needs of the Schoolfield population in that workers had no one to care for them since they had left extended family behind in Appalachia.[58] Not only was there a need for sick care among workers and their families, but also health promotion and education.

Under Hylton's leadership, the welfare program flourished. By 1913 the mill village was situated on the mill compound of 1,600 acres that included 500 houses and a population 4,500 inhabitants.[59] The Dan River Mills owners were proud of their healthy and "ideal" Schoolfield Village community, touting that even the location of the mill, in a hilly area, afforded perfect drainage and each mill home had private, well-built sanitary privies.[60]

Culture played a significant role in how some mill families initially accepted the individuals who provided the company's welfare services. The rural values of self-reliance, combined with their loss of community as they knew it, led many families to mistrust and challenge the new ways of life that the welfare programs were attempting to provide for them. Thus, the nurses invested a great deal of time and effort to gain the trust of transplanted mill workers.[61]

All of the nurses resided in the Schoolfield mill village. In order for the nurses to build trust in the mill village it was important that they live among the workers and take part in village social events. Acceptance into the mill village culture helped open the door for extended welfare services. The mill nurses became intermediaries between the employer and employee and maintained high morale in the mill village through their professionalism and caring practice. It was through these relationships that nurses were able to encourage more workers to utilize the company health care and welfare services available. Often under the guise of making a social call, the nurses visited mill families in their homes. These visits, in addition to participating in village entertainment and social activities, also helped to gain the trust of the mill town citizens.

The industrial nurses' work was varied and stretched their professional training and skills on a daily basis. Each nurse kept clinic hours and received Monday afternoons off. The head nurse received a salary of $50 per month. The nurses were on call at all hours of the day and night.[62]

Like other industrial nurses, the nurses in Schoolfield made home visits to mill workers and their families. In addition to their visiting duties, the nurses of Dan River Mills assisted in an ear, nose, and throat clinic with an average of 25 patients each week. These clinics resulted in three to five surgeries each month to remove adenoids and tonsils in mill children. Under the mill's welfare program, all clinic and surgical services were fully furnished by the mill. Mill nurses also inspected school-age children and children at the Mill's Day Nursery for contagious disease and illness.

Nurses were attentive to the needs of both permanent and temporary mill workers. Transient mill workers who experienced the welfare departments of several southern mills actually became somewhat of authorities on which mills provided the best care. The nurses gained popularity and their services were utilized based on similar experiences throughout the mill villages. Word of mouth and visibility became the nurses' own personal advertisement in the close-knit network of southern mill villages. The transient workers played an active part in spreading the word to smaller mills about industrial welfare programs. The news of healthy workers and successful mill towns gave other mill owners the incentive to improve benefits at their own sites in order to retain more workers.[63]

In a 1919 Red Cross survey, Dan River Mills was reported to be the only plant in the area that provided advanced and successful welfare work. The same survey noted that collaboration between the local community and the mill village was evident in the support provided by several visiting nurses from the Danville, Virginia. Further collaboration and recognition of the welfare program's success is evident by the Ministering Circle of Kings

Daughters benevolent society, and the Metropolitan Life Insurance Company's monetary contributions to Riverside Cotton Mills nurses' salaries and the maintenance of a horse and buggy for their visits.[64]

CONCLUSION

The paternalistic character of early southern industries toward their workers is important to the history of public welfare. Nurses played an integral role in southern mill villages' welfare programs during the early 20th century. The nurses broke through many social, economic, professional, and gender barriers as they established their significance in many mill companies' welfare programs.

The visiting nurses established a rapport with the workers and represented the foundation for access to care within cotton mill villages. Despite some cultural challenges, the services provided by the nurses were soon appreciated by the mill workers. Resourcefulness and collaborative relationships became key to successfully meeting the needs of the mill village residents. In addition to the success experienced by the nurses and workers, company owners whose mills employed nurses came to realize that the move was both successful and an economical approach to meeting increasingly more stringent labor regulations and at the same time gained workers' loyalty. Well-trained mill nurses also possessed the necessary in-depth knowledge of their respective companies and current labor regulations; such knowledge was crucial to the nurses as they made appropriate safety recommendations for their mills. The industrial nurse was available to all employees and collaborated with fellow welfare workers to encourage healthy habits and prevent injury and disease. The relationships between mill owners, workers, and nurses served as a foundation for successful welfare services in industrial villages.

Economics, society, and health were affected by the industrialization of the South in both positive and negative ways. The availability of jobs and resources unknown on the rural farm enabled many poor farmers to rise in social class. However, the resettlement of many rural families presented the health problems similar to crowding in urban cities. Health suffered due to the transition to village life and the effects of industrial work. In the first part of the century, industrial nursing, like many aspects of public health at the time, focused its efforts on sanitation and education practices to improve the health of the community. Riverside Cotton Mills in Schoolfield, Virginia, illustrates how large industrial welfare programs and local and regional health programs collaborated in the early 20th-century South to prevent illness and improve the health of workers and the community.

NOTES

1. Hattie Hylton, *Schoolfield Work Work-Aims, Methods, and Results* (Presented at the Welfare Conference of Southern Employers: Black Mountain, North Carolina, July 16, 1915), 3.

2. Hattie Hylton, *Schoolfield Work*, 3.

3. Lillian Wald, "The Doctor and the Nurse in Industrial Establishments," *The American Journal of Nursing* 12, no. 5 (February 1912): 403–408.

4. Wald's nurses were not the first nurses in industry. As early as 1878 nurses worked in industrial settings in Great Britain. The first American nurse to work for a company was Ada Stewart at the Vermont Marble Company. Wald's work solidified the practice of public health nurses in industry as a specialty.

5. Karen Buhler-Wilkerson, *No Place Like Home* (Baltimore, MD: Johns Hopkins University Press, 2001), 148.

6. Lillian D. Wald, *The House on Henry Street* (New York, NY: Henry Holt, 1915), 208.

7. Buhler-Wilkerson, *No Place Like Home*, 109.

8. Buhler-Wilkerson, *No Place Like Home*, 110.

9. In order to meet the high demands of industrial work, nurses looked to the National Organization of Public Health Nursing (NOPHN) for professional leadership and standards of practice, and met the same professional education standards as public health nurses, which included 3 to 6 months of postgraduate didactic and practicum training at visiting nurses associations. Industrialists expected the same training and expert knowledge when hiring nurses in the South. This education readied the nurses to care for industrial workers and their families in southern cotton mills.

10. Arlene Keeling, *Nursing and the Privilege of Prescription, 1893–2000* (Columbus, OH: Ohio State University Press, 2007), 25.

11. Virginia's Piedmont region extends from Danville in southeast Virginia into northern North Carolina.

12. Jennings Jefferson Rhyne, *Some Southern Cotton Mill Workers and Their Villages* (Chapel Hill, NC: University of North Carolina Press, 1930).

13. Spindles are machines used to spin raw cotton into thread.

14. Robert King, *Robert Addison Schoolfield (1853–1931): A Biographical History of the Leader of Danville, Virginia, Textile Mills During the First 50 Years* (Richmond, VA: William Byrd Press, 1979), 55.

15. Jacquelyn Dowd Hall et al., *Like a Family: The Making of a Southern Cotton Mill World* (Chapel Hill, NC: University of North Carolina Press, 1987), 3-7.

16. Hall et al., *Like a Family*, 8.

17. Hall et al., *Like a Family*, 5–9.

18. Melton McLaurin, *Paternalism and Protest: Southern Cotton Mill Workers and Organized Labor, 1875–1905* (Westport, CT: Negro Universities Press, 1971), 12.

19. Edward Beardsley, *A History of Neglect: Health Care for Blacks and Mill Workers in the Twentieth-Century South* (Knoxville, TN: University of Tennessee Press, 1987), 42.

20. By 1877, reconstruction was ending and politicians began to take back power in the southern states. Proposed legislation known as Jim Crow laws, nicknamed after a derogatory set of plays depicting Blacks, aimed to segregate by race, employment, social events, housing, and education. Literacy tests, poll taxes, and voter registration disenfranchised Black men from voting. In 1896 the United States Supreme Court case *Plessy vs. Ferguson*, a dispute over the segregation of passenger train cars in New Orleans, ruled that facilities separated by race did not violate the Constitution if the facilities were equal. Essentially, the Supreme Court ruled segregation was not discrimination. Equal but separate cultural norms were solidified by law and full rights of citizenship in America were denied to Blacks.

21. McLaurin, *Paternalism and Protest*, 12.

22. American Red Cross Report: Red Cross Survey of Danville Virginia, 1919 (National Archives College Park Maryland, box 572, File 509.1).

23. American Red Cross Report, 1919.

24. Harriet L. Herring, *Welfare Work in Mill Villages* (Chapel Hill, NC: University of North Carolina Press, 1929), 163-167.

25. Herring, *Welfare Work in Mill Villages*, 165.

26. Hall et al., *Like a Family*, 93.

27. Beardsley, *A History of Neglect*, 63–64.

28. Beardsley, *A History of Neglect*, 64–67.

29. Hall et al., *Like a Family*, 93.

30. Hall et al., *Like a Family*, 81–82.

31. Hall et al., *Like a Family*, 81–82.

32. Beardsley, *A History of Neglect*, 189–190.

33. Beardsley, *A History of Neglect*. Pellagra is the result of profound niacin deficiency and often associated with malnutrition; characterized by cutaneous, gastrointestinal, mucosal, and neurological symptoms. *Taber's A Cyclopedic Medical Dictionary*, ed. Donald Venes, 20th ed. (Philadelphia, PA: F. A. Davis, 2005), 54-56.

34. Beardsley, *A History of Neglect*, 56.

35. Beardsley, *A History of Neglect*, 189.

36. Herring, *Welfare Work in Mill Villages*, 161.

37. Herring, *Welfare Work in Mill Villages*, 161.

38. Florence Swift Wright, *Industrial Nursing* (New York, NY: Cornell Press, 1920), 27.

39. Lillian Wald Papers, Council of National Defense correspondence, Lillian Wald Papers, New York Public Library, microfilm, reel 25.

40. Herring, *Welfare Work in Mill Villages*, 167.

41. Wilhelmina A. Carver, "The Field of Industrial Nursing: What the Student Nurse Should Know About It," *The American Journal of Nursing* 30, no. 9 (September 1930): 1114–18.

42. Wright, *Industrial Nursing,* 47.

43. Wright, *Industrial Nursing,* 28-29.

44. Workmen's compensation was a form of injury and accident compensation established in the industrialized nations of Great Britain and Germany in the late 1890s. The legislation in those two countries not only placed the responsibility of compensation for industrial accidents and death on the employer, but also instituted regulations to make the workplace safer. The 1908 compensation laws for federal workers paved the way for workmen's compensation legislation. However, workmen's compensation legislation was not compulsory. Instead each state created and passed some type of workmen's compensation between 1909 and 1948. Virginia adopted a version of workmen's compensation legislation in January 1918. The law ultimately placed the responsibility and the cost of job-related injury on the employer. The content and implementation of labor legislation varied from state to state.

45. Wright, *Industrial Nursing,* 54.

46. Wright, *Industrial Nursing,* 48–49.

47. Herring, *Welfare Work in Mill Villages,* 129–30.

48. Herring, *Welfare Work in Mill Villages,* 130.

49. Herring, *Welfare Work in Mill Villages,* 130.

50. Carver, "Field of Industrial Nursing," 1116.

51. Herring, *Welfare Work in Mill Villages.*

52. Patricia D' Antonio, *American Nursing: A History of Knowledge, Authority, and the Meaning of Work* (Baltimore, MD: Johns Hopkins University Press, 2010), 122–127.

53. King, *Robert Addison Schoolfield,* 55.

54. *The Mill News* 22, no. 1 (October 14, 1920).

55. Andrea Tone, *The Business of Benevolence* (Ithaca, NY: Cornell University Press, 1997), 33–35.

56. Tone, *Business of Benevolence,* 43.

57. Hylton, *Schoolfield Work,* 3.

58. Robert Sidney Smith, *Mill on the Dan* (1960), 108.

59. King, *Robert Addison Schoolfield,* 68-69.

60. King, *Robert Addison Schoolfield,* 2–3.

61. Herring, *Welfare Work in Mill Villages,* 167.

62. Pearl Wyche, correspondence to Moses and Ceasar Cone, June 1913, Southern Historical Collection, Wilson Library, University of Chapel Hill, Chapel Hill, NC. Cone Mills Corporate Records box 122, Folder 1240.

63. American Red Cross Report, 1919, 3–4.

64. American Red Cross Report, 1919, 65.

5

•••••

Care in the Coal Fields: Promoting Health Through Sanitation and Nutrition

•••••

JOHN C. KIRCHGESSNER

We began with a liquid diet consisting largely of buttermilk and juices each hour while awake, and water between. As they improved, soft foods were added.[1]

EVA MCKEAN PROVIDED THESE STANDARD instructions to those caring for the sick during a typhoid epidemic in the 1930s. As the only nurse in one West Virginia coal camp, she regularly gave care instructions to the family members and moved on to others. Provided with a car and gasoline, and a wage for merely 1 month, McKean provided care to the camp's 30 typhoid victims. Relying on her training and education, as well as her previous experience working in coal camps, she devised a plan of care to make the best use of her time and resources. She made frequent home visits and educated one family member on how to take a temperature, how to bathe the patient to reduce high fevers, and how to keep meticulous records. In addition, she instructed family members to provide the strict diet described above—a necessity for all patients recovering from typhoid. Despite geographic barriers and limited access to other modern health care, McKean's professional expertise and skills, as well as her experience in providing care in remote rural settings, resulted in the full recovery of all 30 patients.[2] Eva McKean's success in providing care to the typhoid victims testifies how nurses, despite barriers to care and limited resources, were able to provide professional nursing care in the mountainous and isolating terrain in West Virginia's coal fields.

FROM MOUNTAINEERS TO MINERS

During the post–Civil War era, labor migrations from the southern United States and Europe transformed the state of West Virginia. The state's rich natural resources including bituminous coal led to the development of some of America's largest industries. Coal became the sole source of fuel for the American railroad and shipping industries. As well, it was the only source of energy to produce electricity, iron, and steel, all of which were used to build many of America's major cities during the late-19th and early-20th centuries. By 1907 West Virginia had moved from a predominantly agrarian–mountaineering culture comprised of native-born Americans to an urban–industrialized culture in touch with the world. And yet, despite the state's connections to the world economy, West Virginia remained a mountainous state with roots deeply embedded in Appalachian culture. For many of its citizens, access to modern health care remained a challenge due to geographic, economic, and cultural barriers.

While the health care concerns associated with mining disasters and catastrophic injuries were well publicized and visible, most of the basic health care concerns in the coal mining towns remained invisible, unknown, and uncared for. The Department of Public Health in West Virginia faced the issues of poor sanitation, inadequate housing, and lack of maternal–child health care. However, as in many regions across the country, the Department of Public Health was overburdened and understaffed. Thus, many of these concerns were not addressed adequately and the miners and their families suffered the consequences. As a result, plans to meet the health care needs in the mining towns became a patchwork quilt of sorts. Public health officials, nurses, local physicians, coal company doctors, and the coal industry itself pieced together the variety of necessary services to decrease the mortality and morbidity caused by inadequate health care.

COAL COMPANY CARE

Coal was first discovered in West Virginia in 1742.[3] As the coal industry grew throughout the 19th and early 20th centuries, the health care needs of the West Virginia coal miners and their families became more complex. The early coal camps, often quickly established and containing no more than tents and crudely constructed shanties, housed mostly men. Eventually the wives and families began to join the miners and they required better shelter and more organized towns. Thus, the management of the coal companies established towns near the mines and provided essential services: medicine, housing, electricity, water, sewage, schools, and a general store—the "company store."

The quality of these essentials varied from coal town to coal town, depending on the philosophy and compassion of the owner of the local mine. Capitalistic paternalism was the driving force that dictated how coal-company owners approached managing the mine and the men and boys who extracted it. The disparity in the philosophies of caring among coal company owners resulted in great differences in housing conditions and the quality of public services found in the coal towns throughout the region. For example, the Stonega Coke and Coal Company referred to its paternalism as "contentment sociology," which included health care.[4] This coal company provided housing and other town services to keep miners on the job and as productive as possible while generating additional income for the company. They also used their "contentment sociology" as a recruitment and retention strategy.[5]

Unlike the mines found in the anthracite coal regions of Pennsylvania, few mines in West Virginia were near cities or even incorporated towns that had housing, supplies, and health care readily available.[6] Until the early 20th century, the health care provided to West Virginia miners and their families was generally in the form of the "company doctor," a system that prevailed into the first half of the century.[7] As implied by his title, the coal company doctor was hired and paid by the company running the mine. Since no standards were in place, the qualification of these physicians varied greatly. The company doctor had a wide variety of responsibilities and played many roles: town sanitarian supervisor, public health officer, surgeon, and obstetrician, to name a few. For quite some time the company doctor system worked; but as the coal mining industry became modernized and mines became larger, the number of traumatic injuries multiplied and the number of people in the towns increased. Many company doctors realized that they could not provide all of the health care services required of them. One physician per town was no longer a viable system for care.

HEALTH CARE ABOVEGROUND AND UNDERGROUND

Throughout the Progressive Era of the early 20th century (1900–1918), state and federal agencies focused on addressing and curing the many social ills in American society. One of these was the poor conditions prevalent in coal mines and their nearby towns. Since mine safety and miners' injuries were continually in the forefront of health care concerns throughout the era, both the state and federal governments established new policies to create safer working conditions for coal miners.[8] This certainly was progress, but state and national boards of health were equally concerned about the sanitation issues inside the mines. As a result the board leaders began to put policies in place to enforce mine health and sanitary codes.[9]

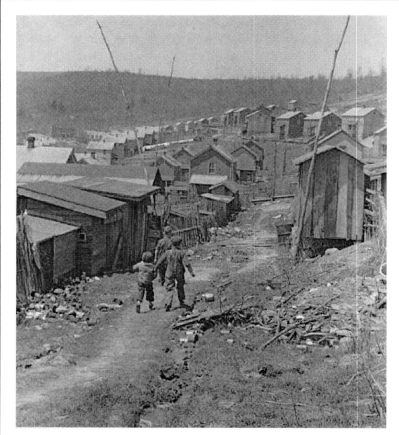

Crowded housing in company-owned coal town.

• • • • •

While health conditions were poor underground, they were in some cases dire aboveground. Sanitation, epidemics, housing, refuse removal, and polluted water were some of the health and sanitation issues that continually vexed coal company operators and public health officials.[10] Eventually the combination of government pressure and welfare capitalism persuaded more mine owners to address the social ills that plagued their towns. In 1913, the Tennessee Coal and Iron Company established its own health department that included dispensaries and small emergency hospitals.[11] In 1916, the Stonega Coke and Coal Company hired nurses who placed greater emphasis on the prevention of infectious diseases.[12]

By 1920 both companies began to embrace the relatively new specialty of industrial medicine. In so doing, coal company operators began to recognize, and even admit, that the company doctor system was no longer keeping its employees content, healthy, and productive.[13] However, historian Claude Shifflett notes, "Altruism seldom motivated the operators to provide social institutions . . . good health care or comfortable homes. . . . Labor expediency in a labor-short market, together with the financial security of operating a company set the boundaries for paternalism. Operators believed that paternalism was just another cost of doing business."[14] Whether the West Virginia coal companies provided services and benefits to their miners out of altruism, benevolence, a need for financial stability, or a combination of all three, the companies' benefits were simply not enough to support a healthy population and a work force among the state's coal towns.

Throughout the Progressive Era, public health became an important cause for policy makers, social activists, physicians, and nurses. With knowledge of the advancements in science and medicine, physicians and nurses alike better understood the etiology of many common infectious diseases. But despite a better understanding, the mortality and morbidity rates in many urban and rural areas remained high. Lillian Wald, a pioneer in public health care nursing in New York City's Lower East Side, daily addressed the health care needs of citizens who often did not have a voice in society. Wald envisioned a collaborative professional model for health care, one in which nurses were the first line of care and physicians cared for complex patients. In this model, nurses practiced to the full extent of their knowledge and training. Wald also envisioned this model as ideal to care for industrial workers, a group known to be often socially disenfranchised and medically underserved.[15] Some manufacturing industries had already begun to employ nurses and Wald noted in 1912 that, "Nurses are required to assist the factory surgeons and to take general care of the girls, assisting them to regulate their diet and personal hygiene, caring for them when they suffer from vague symptoms of fatigue, over-strain and bad air."[16] Wald went on to further encourage all industrial employees to expect and maintain safe health conditions. She also stressed the need for the public to promote policy that would insist on supervision and education for better health and safety practices in America's factories.[17]

Commenting on the conditions in the Appalachian region in the 1920s, historian Sandra Lee Barney notes, "Sanitation, nutrition, and hygiene issues were of the most immediate concern among coal miners and other industrial workers."[18] But due to the lack of resources and a well-developed public health infrastructure, the health care and social needs of West Virginia's citizens needed to be addressed by many different groups that were committed to improving the health of the state's general population and its workers. In some regions throughout Appalachia, middle-class elite women's groups, club women, and settlement workers joined forces with physicians. These groups of women were known for hiring public health nurses to educate families and screen women and children for common illnesses; in so doing, the health of many miners and their families slowly began to improve.[19]

But despite these collaborative efforts, health care continued to lag behind in rural West Virginia. In 1923 the U.S. Children's Bureau published its report on the lives of children in the West Virginian coal fields. The report recorded that the living conditions of 645 families, including 1,965 children, was generally substandard. The report concluded that the paternalistic policies of the coal companies were at fault, noting, "Whether conditions are good or bad depends upon the policy of the coal company and not upon the will of the inhabitants."[20] The Bureaus report also noted that in some towns the residents' privies emptied directly into the creeks that provided water to the towns. In other towns, the residents allowed their farm animals to roam free; their animals' waste further added to the sanitation hazards. Housing conditions varied widely from town to town and was often substandard, both in size and quality.[21]

All of these factors contributed to the town residents' well-being or lack thereof. Many illnesses that plagued the miners and their families, including typhoid fever, were triggered by poor living conditions. The Bureau noted in its report, however, that coal towns in which the quality of life was excellent had well-maintained, painted houses, well-kept yards and roads, and lighted streets.[22] The Bureau report also noted that only one public health

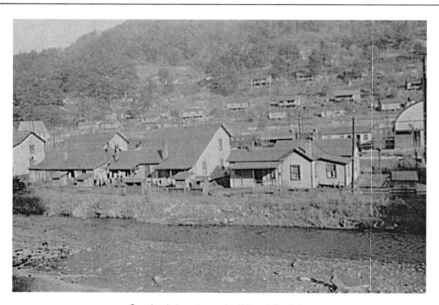

Coal mining town in West Virginia.

● ● ● ● ●

nurse provided care to miners in two coal camps.[23] The lack of professional resources greatly hampered access to health care.

The incidence of childhood illnesses, such as measles, whooping cough, and diphtheria, was reported to be higher among children living in the West Virginia coal fields than children living in the coal towns of Pennsylvania. Influenza, tuberculosis, rheumatism, and disabilities related to childbirth were also prevalent among miner's wives. The illness plaguing both mothers and children were related to the quality of their living conditions.[24] Infant and maternal mortality rates were high throughout many of the coal towns in West Virginia.[25] These statistics are evidence that despite the efforts of company doctors, and the establishment of state miners' hospitals in 1901, the health care needs of mining communities were not being met; the need for a stronger public health presence was crucial.

NURSES IN THE COAL FIELDS

As early as 1888, coal companies employed nurses in the anthracite coal region of Pennsylvania. One group of companies hired Betty Moulder in 1888 to care for the miners and their families.[26] This fact and information about the nurses who worked in the West Virginia miners' hospitals are almost all that is mentioned in the literature or in archival material regarding nurses in the coal fields before the 1930s. There is, however, one exception. One coal company did provide professional care to its miners in the 1920s prior to the Great Depression. The Consolidated Coal Company employed several coal camp nurses. Eva Ruth McKean, a West Virginia native, was one of the nurses hired by the company. McKean's duties were to assist the company doctors on a daily basis, conduct monthly health classes in the camp's schools, teach first aid, and inspect all of the school children for health problems.[27] As part of her work in the company's prenatal clinics, McKean was required to visit the expectant mothers, provide basic childbirth education once a month, and make sure all the necessary provisions were available for home deliveries. Also included in her role as coal camp nurse, McKean accompanied the camp superintendent and physicians on periodic tours of the camp to observe sanitation conditions. If the group noted any problems, McKean was responsible to follow up by visiting the families and advising them on how to improve the conditions at their residences.[28] In McKean's words, "There were few injuries at the mine and [they] were seen only by the doctor. . . . Since prevention of disease was highly stressed, I did very little active nursing while with this company."[29] Unfortunately, as the Great Depression descended on the nation, industrial productivity came to a halt, the once high quantity of coal declined, and West Virginia's coal mines produced fewer tons per year. Consolidated Coal profits declined and the nursing service became another casualty of the Great Depression.[30]

KOPPERS NURSES IMPROVE ACCESS TO CARE

Not all nursing services were suspended during the Great Depression, however. During the peak of the Depression, the Koppers Coal Division of Eastern Gas and Fuel Associates of Boston established a nursing service. Founded in 1934 and known as the Koppers Coal Nursing Service, it was described by its assistant supervisor Ruby Thompson Shirey as, ". . . a kind of public health nursing which includes school, child and maternal health, and industrial nursing."[31] All of the nurses were residents of West Virginia and, therefore, understood the needs of the miners and their families. Perhaps even of more importance was the fact that these nurses understood the mining culture, and thus were generally well accepted by the community. As a result of their hiring native-born West Virginians, the Koppers Coal Division was able to overcome a barrier often associated with a lack of cultural access to care. In spite of overcoming one barrier, another still remained. The local and company physicians, who did not understand the extent of the care that the Koppers nurses could provide, had to be convinced that the nurses' services were vital to the communities they served.

The West Virginia Health Department, however, was very cooperative with the plan for a nursing service. Ruby Shirey noted, "The West Virginia Public Health Department feels that our nurses relieve them of many duties which they would not be able to handle, as this department is greatly overworked."[32] The Koppers nurses placed a great deal of emphasis on education and prevention and, like Eva McKean, they helped to educate entire families, while focusing on the mothers and children. The education included first aid classes and home hygiene. Through these classes, the nurses ultimately provided the women in the communities with the knowledge and skills that allowed them to care for each other during illness, childbirth, and confinement. As Ruby Shirey noted, these skills were vital since private-duty nurses were not readily available in the coal fields and financially out of reach for most miners.[33] The nurses assisted in prenatal clinics, keeping careful records of each woman's progress and attending to the mother at delivery. Shirey further noted that, "During delivery, she assists the doctor and if there is any need for anesthesia or the repair of lacerations, she can put her knowledge of surgical nursing to good use."[34] Their diverse responsibilities and activities clearly show that the nurses were practicing to the full extent of their education and training.

Making visits, educating women, and participating in deliveries were just some of the nurses' roles. In addition to these various responsibilities, the nurses set aside a part of each day for office hours. During this office time the nurses assisted the physicians, dressed injuries, and followed up on paperwork; by assisting with office visits, the nurses were able to stay abreast of the illnesses and accidents that occurred in the community and take appropriate action.

Providing postpartum care was responsibility of the nurses. During each mother's postpartum period, the nurses visited the mother and infant every day. In their concern for the baby's well-being, they weighed the infant weekly for a month, then monthly for the first year. Their assessment skills and professional judgment were essential during these visits. Based on the infant's weight, the nurses made dietary recommendations to the mother and advised that cod liver oil be given daily.[35] After the first year of a child's life, the nurses continued to follow the children's progress, seeing them once a year in a preschool clinic. During the clinic checkup they examined the children and administered the necessary immunizations. If they detected any "defects" during the visit to the clinic, the nurses made follow-up visits to the children's homes and discussed any plans with the mothers for addressing their children's needs. Once the children were of school age, the nurses continued their care through frequent school visits. With each visit the nurses reviewed the children's immunization records and recorded the children's height and weight. Once a month nurses weighed the children; once every 3 months they measured the children's height. For those children who were underweight and/or in the first through fourth grades, nurses advised the parents to give the children a daily dose of cod liver oil from October to April. Nurses also made sure that any underweight children received hot lunches during the school day to provide extra calories and nutrition.

In the 1930s, the nurses extended their monitoring of the nutritional status of school children to include whole families living in the coal mining community. As the Great Depression continued and the nation's economic conditions declined, the productivity of the Koppers coal mines declined as well. Less demand for coal meant less work and ultimately less income for the miners. These worsening economic conditions caused great concern among the Koppers nurses as they witnessed an increase in hunger and malnutrition among the coal mining families. In order to better assess and monitor the nutritional status of the miners and their families, the nurses made frequent home visits to instruct and assist mothers in providing healthy meals that were within their families' limited means.

The nurses' nutritional counseling never ended. The economic problems created by the low income of the coal miners in the depression years changed over to a food scarcity problem beginning in the early 1940s. As World War II encompassed the United States, essential foods became scarce through the need for rationing. The nurses continued their nutritional education program through a campaign known as "Koppers Health for Victory Clubs." The Victory Clubs involved all the families and provided the nurses the opportunity to educate them on good nutrition and to demonstrate how to prepare healthy meals from the food that was available.

The expert and well-organized care provided by the Koppers nurses during the first 10 years of existence is noteworthy. From 1936 to 1944 the death rate among children from birth to 14 years of age was reduced by 50%; the number of abortions, miscarriages, and still births was reduced as well. These findings were attributed to the care and education the families received from the nurses in the prenatal and preschool clinics and from the frequent home visits. In many of the coal-town schools, immunization rates were almost at 100%, thus reducing the incidence of typhoid, diphtheria, and small pox. School absences from common ailments such as colds were reduced as well, and it was believed at the time that this was the result of the nurses' liberal use of cod liver oil.[36]

CONCLUSION

In the first half of the 20th century, the infrastructure of the United States focused on the need for public health and sanitation. Although this focus contributed directly to the modernization of U.S. towns and cities in most areas, the remote rural towns of West Virginia struggled to provide improved services to their citizens. Like many other departments of health in rural states, the West Virginia Department of Health lacked the professional resources necessary to keep the state's general population healthy. The advent of modern coal mining in West Virginia and the resulting expanded population left the state unable to keep up with the demands necessary for quality public health. Thus, the Department of Health relied on multiple sources of public health care, sources that included local and regional women's groups, company physicians, the state's miners' hospitals, and nurses. Nurses were instrumental in addressing and managing the public health care needs of both the general public and the coal miners. By practicing to the full extent of their training and using their experience and ingenuity, they overcame many of the barriers to care, namely geography, economic means, and culture to slowly improve the health of miners and their families.

Some coal companies provided more extensive health care services for miners and their families beyond a single company physician. These companies provided for the medical welfare of their miners by employing nurses who, in turn, provided care to women and children as well as education in health, nutrition, and sanitation. Using the models of public health and industrial health prescribed by Lillian Wald, the Koppers nurses brought professional nursing resources to the coal fields. Daily they assessed, diagnosed, advised, made critical decisions, and recommended care and comfort to their patients and their families. The Koppers Coal Nursing Service illustrates how one industry and one state attempted to address the often daunting task of meeting so many health care needs of so many people; people often denied geographic, economic, and cultural access to care. The nursing service also illustrates how nurses in rural areas, decades before advanced practice nurses existed, used their knowledge, experience, and skills to practice to the full extent of their education.

NOTES

1. Ruby Shirey, "Nursing Miners and Their Families: The Koppers Coal Nursing Service," *The American Journal of Nursing* 44 (April 1944): 347.

2. Claude Frazier, *Miners and Medicine: West Virginia Memories* (Norman, OK: University of Oklahoma Press, 1992), 103.

3. Office of MHS&T, "West Virginia Office of Miners' Health Safety and Training: A Brief History of Coal and Health and Safety Enforcement in West Virginia," http://www.wvminesafety.org/History.htm. paragraph 2.

4. Crandall A. Shifflett. *Coal Towns: Life, Work, and Culture in Company Town of Southern Appalachia, 1880–1960* (Knoxville, TN: The University of Tennessee Press, 1991), 54.

5. Shifflett, *Coal Towns*, 54.

6. Many of the anthracite coal towns in Pennsylvania were clustered along rivers and streams. In addition, railroads, good roads, and telephone service allowed communication and aided in continuous contact with others. In 1923, "70 per cent of the anthracite mine workers live in incorporated towns of 2,500 population or over . . . 90 per cent of the men live in houses not owned by the coal companies." Marie L. Obenauer, "The Price of Coal. Anthracite and Bituminous," *Annals of the American Academy of Political and Social Science*, vol. 111 (Philadelphia, PA: American Academy of Political and Social Science, January 1924), 22.

7. Despite being the coal company owners, system of choice, it was recognized by the early 1900s that company doctors were often ill prepared, both educationally and logistically, to care for the increasingly devastating injuries that were occurring inside the mines; no longer could surgeries be performed in the physicians' offices or the miners' homes. This concern ultimately led to the establishment of the West Virginia miners' hospitals in 1899. Thus, organized medical and nursing care was provided to miners. However, the need for coal company doctors would continue throughout the next 50 years. John C. Kirchgessner, "The Miners' Hospitals of West Virginia: Nurses and Healthcare Come to the Coal Fields, 1900–1920," *Nursing History Review* 8 (2000): 157–168.

8. http://www.wvminesafety.org/History.htm. West Virginia hired its first mine inspector in 1883 and mine safety began to be addressed in state policy with the first comprehensive mine safety laws proposed in 1884. The U.S. Bureau of Mines was established in 1910. Child labor laws also became more stringent in the 1910s, thus helping to curtail the tragedies that occurred to children working in West Virginia mines.

9. Medical historian Claude Frazier notes, "Sanitation in the mines presented a nasty problem . . . Excreta and litter accumulated, and rats frequently found a haven in the muck. . . ." Claude Frazier, *Miners and Medicine: West Virginia Memories* (Norman, OK: University of Oklahoma Press, 1992), 33.

10. Shifflett, *Coal Towns*, 56.

11. Shifflett, *Coal Towns*, 55.

12. Shifflett, *Coal Towns*, 55.

13. Shifflett, *Coal Towns*, 55.

14. Shifflett, *Coal Towns*, 66.

15. Lillian Wald, "The Doctor and the Nurse in Industrial Establishments," *The American Journal of Nursing* 12, no. 5 (February 1912): 403–408.

16. Wald, "The Doctor and the Nurse in Industrial Establishments," 407.

17. Wald, "The Doctor and the Nurse in Industrial Establishments," 407.

18. Sandra Barney, *Authorized to Heal: Gender, Class, and the Transformation of Medicine in Appalachia, 1880–1930* (Chapel Hill, NC: The University of North Carolina Press, 2000), 101. In addition, Barney notes that, "Appalachian miners and their families suffered exceptionally high rates of typhoid, scarlet fever, tuberculosis, and diphtheria," p. 104.

19. Barney, *Authorized to Heal*, 100–104.

20. Nettie McGill, "The Welfare of Children in Bituminous Coal Mining Communities in West Virginia," *U.S. Department of Labor, Children's Bureau* (Washington, DC: Washington Government Printing Office, 1923), 7, 11.

21. McGill, "Welfare of Children." McGill notes that the water sources for towns varied greatly and ranged from creeks, hydrants, shallow wells, and cisterns with many creeks and springs "contaminated by chickens . . . by dishwater, drainage, and garbage" p. 15; Price Fishback and Dieter Lauszus, "The Quality of Services in Company Towns: Sanitation in Coal Towns During the 1920s," *The Journal of Economic History* 49, no. 1 (March 1989): 125–44; Barney, *Authorized to Heal*, 104.

22. McGill, "Welfare of Children," 10.

23. McGill, "Welfare of Children," 50.

24. McGill, "Welfare of Children," 47.

25. McGill, "Welfare of Children," 50–52. Facts regarding infant mortality rates among coal mining families were found to be poorly recorded. However, the infant mortality rates in the coal towns surveyed were estimated in 1923 to be 94 per 1000 infants born alive; this statistic was above the 1915–1920 national average for rural areas, p. 51.

26. "Short History of Industrial Nursing by the American Association of Industrial Nurses," 1976: 1.

27. Frazier, *Miners and Medicine,* 102.

28. Frazier, *Miners and Medicine,* 102.

29. Frazier, *Miners and Medicine,* 103.

30. Frazier, *Miners and Medicine,* 103.

31. Shirey, "Nursing Miners and Their Families," 347.

32. Shirey, "Nursing Miners and Their Families," 347.

33. Shirey, "Nursing Miners and Their Families," 348.

34. Shirey, "Nursing Miners and Their Families," 348.

35. Shirey, "Nursing Miners and Their Families," 348.

36. Shirey, "Nursing Miners and Their Families," 348.

6

•••••

Mary Breckinridge and the Frontier Nursing Service: Saddlebags and Swinging Bridges

•••••

ANNE Z. COCKERHAM

The principle of organization in a remotely rural field of work is one of *decentralization*. In such a country, *time* and not mileage is the factor involved in daily travel and in all emergencies. It is not a question of the patient's distance from his nurse but of how long it takes her to reach him. This is as true of travel by dogsled in the Labrador snows or travel by boat in the Outer Hebrides, as it is in the Kentucky mountains. It is the crux of the problem to be handled . . . After nurse–midwives were stationed at all of the six outpost nursing centers of the Frontier Nursing Service . . . we covered an area of approximately 700 square miles in which we carried bedside nursing, midwifery, and public health to nearly 10,000 people. Our aim [was to leave] no territory uncovered and no people uncared for.[1]

WRITING IN HER AUTOBIOGRAPHY, *Wide Neighborhoods*, nurse and midwife Mary Breckinridge described the organizing principles of her rural Frontier Nursing Service (FNS) in Eastern Kentucky. This decentralized system allowed the residents of the remote and mountainous service area to benefit from nurses' acute and preventive care for general medical and obstetrical needs. Riding on horseback with their supplies in saddlebags and sometimes crossing creek beds on swinging bridges to reach remote cabins, FNS nurses provided access to health care for thousands of mountain people between 1925 and the 1950s.

ROOTS OF THE FRONTIER NURSING SERVICE

Mary Breckinridge's rich and varied professional and personal experiences, dedication, and vision culminated in the founding of the Frontier Nursing Service. Born into a wealthy, politically well-connected, and public service-oriented Southern family,[2] Breckinridge longed to contribute to society in a more far-reaching way than was typical of women in her social group in the early 20th century.[3] She chose trained nursing and developed what would become a lifelong affinity to care for the most vulnerable members of society—mothers and their children.

After a series of painful life events that included widowhood, divorce, and the deaths of her two beloved young children, Breckinridge redoubled her commitment to maternal–child health.[4] In 1918 Breckinridge traveled as a lecturer for the United States Children's Bureau and gained a keen appreciation for the plight of rural American children.[5] Later, through her nursing work in rural areas in post-Great War France as part of the Comité Américain pour les Régions Dévastées de le France (CARD, the American Committee for Devastated France), Breckinridge gained valuable insights not only about organizational dynamics, but also about strategies for accomplishing complex and difficult missions in remote environments.[6] Indeed, Breckinridge's experiences in the United States and abroad taught her that much had been done to help urban mothers and babies during the Progressive Era years of 1890 to 1920, yet the needs of rural families were great.[7] According to Breckinridge: "Whether in city or country, [children] mattered more to me than all the world beside. But in America, while much had been done for "city children" during the Progressive Era years of 1890 to 1920, "remotely rural children had been neglected."[8]

Breckinridge concluded that she would work for those rural children and that she could best serve them through a maternity care demonstration project. She focused on maternity care because "work for children should begin before they are born, should carry with them through their greatest hazard which is childbirth, and should be most intensive during their first six years of life."[9] Throughout the early 1920s, Breckinridge refined her demonstration project plans and selected a remote area of steep mountains in Eastern Kentucky, an area in which she hoped to capitalize on her deep family roots. It was a part of the country in which "my family name was known and I would be accepted without explanation, because I belonged."[10] Breckinridge's influential family members and close family friends supported her plan. Notably, at least five powerful Kentucky physicians were her cousins. One of these cousins, Waller Bullock, promised Breckinridge, "There isn't one of us, Mary, that won't stand by you."[11]

Eastern Kentucky's remotely rural setting, one of the most isolated and impoverished areas of the United States, accorded credibility to the venture.

According to Breckinridge: "If the work I had in mind could be done there, it could be duplicated anywhere else in the United States with less effort . . . Our inaccessibility was a priceless asset. None who wanted to copy our work could plead that it would be more difficult for them than it had been for us."[12]

Early 20th-century, rural Eastern Kentucky lacked professional medical and nursing care and most mountain women relied on untrained "granny" midwives to attend their births.[13] Moreover, local midwives' attentions centered only on the birth itself and did not include any care during the pregnancy, despite a burgeoning interest in prenatal care as a public health intervention. Complicating matters, few physicians were available to provide either routine or emergency care, and those who were willing to provide care were too far away to help. A Kentucky physician once lamented to Breckinridge that mountain women did not necessarily need more physicians; what birthing women needed were well-trained *professionals* who were geographically well-placed. According to that physician: "It is impossible for me to reach every hoot-owl hollow in my section in time to be of any use to a woman in childbirth. Midwives are essential here. I wish they might be nurses as well."[14]

During the summer of 1923, Breckinridge rode through the mountains of Eastern Kentucky to survey the existing state of midwifery there. On thirteen horses and three mules, Breckinridge rode 650 miles and interviewed 53 granny midwives. These women ranged from what Breckinridge determined to be "intelligent women whose homes were tidy and gay with flowers" to ignorantly superstitious women who were "filthy, as were their homes."[15] The investigation reinforced that a professional nursing service was badly needed. According to Breckinridge, ". . . the care given women in childbirth and their babies, thousands of them in thousands of square miles, was as medieval as the nursing care of the sick in the public hospitals of France."[16]

As her plan for a demonstration project continued to take shape, Breckinridge envisioned that the British model of training in both nursing and midwifery would save the lives of rural mothers and babies. Based on that vision, she then went to England and Scotland to study midwifery practice and education and district nursing. Breckinridge also analyzed the organization of the Highlands and Islands Medical and Nursing Services in Scotland, later using it as a model for the Frontier Nursing Service.[17]

A RURAL NURSE–MIDWIFERY SERVICE IS BORN

Now a trained nurse and midwife, Breckinridge was ready to open her mountain nurse–midwifery service. In May 1925 members of the Kentucky

Committee for Mothers and Babies met. Work moved forward quickly; Breckinridge immediately hired two nurses, and in September 1925, the first clinic opened in Hyden, Kentucky.[18] During the first month, 233 patients made 561 visits to the clinic and the nurses completed 46 home visits.[19] Gradually, more nurses joined the staff, the patient load grew, and the list of facilities expanded. In 1928 Breckinridge changed the organization's name to the Frontier Nursing Service[20] and work was completed on Hyden Hospital, the center of the organization's health care system. By 1929 the service operated six FNS clinics with two more clinics planned.[21]

Soon after she and her nurses had begun their work, Breckinridge realized that although unmet maternity health needs were pressing, general medical and preventive care were equally important; no established systems of preventive or acute health care were accessible to people in Leslie County.[22] Indeed, few physicians were willing to practice in the isolated environment, in cash-poor communities.[23] Consequently, poor health was endemic among mountain people who suffered from dysentery, measles, scarlet fever, whooping cough, tuberculosis, and pneumonia. Mountain children suffered from hookworm and malnutrition; pregnant women were anemic. Mountain men were killed or severely injured while cutting lumber and mining coal. Feuds left opposing family members with gunshot wounds while copperheads and rattlesnakes left mountain people with the devastating consequences of snakebites.[24]

To address general medical needs, Breckinridge soon employed nurses who were *not* midwives and the nurses' first priority was much-needed inoculations. Kentucky Health Commissioner Arthur McCormack had requested the administration of hundreds of typhoid and diphtheria inoculations to combat these endemic illnesses in the mountains. The FNS nurses complied. When they learned of a typhoid outbreak, they traveled to "inoculate the whole creek," riding horseback nearly an entire day to do so.[25] Word of these outbreaks often reached the nurses indirectly. In fact, one time they heard of a diphtheria outbreak through a terrifying report of a baby who "had a risin' in the throat and choked to death." Thus, nursing routines soon included administering toxin-antitoxin injections to every young child in their territory.[26]

As Breckinridge foresaw when she founded the FNS, the mountain people's health needs were immense. Later reflecting on the service's work in those early days, Breckinridge recalled terribly ill children enduring parasitic illnesses typical of rural areas, including "a six-year-old boy with a [hematocrit] of only twenty per cent and skin like parchment, from hookworm." Another child, this one tinier and even more vulnerable, suffered the devastating effects of eye disease: "a four-week-old baby was brought to one of our nursing centers . . . and rushed by the nurse, on horseback, to Hyden Hospital, with both eyes so blinded by pus that it was impossible to tell at first whether any sight could be saved at all." Isolated mountain cabins and transportation challenges added to the difficulties of caring for pregnant women: "More than one expectant mother came in near the end of her pregnancy, and even in labor, riding sideways, on the rump of the horse, behind the nurse–midwife. 'Where else in the world,' we often asked ourselves, 'would a woman be brought to a hospital door in such a fashion?'"[27]

RURAL HEALTH MODEL

Breckinridge wisely considered the unique aspects of a rural setting when she designed the Frontier Nursing Service. The decentralization of the FNS facilities and personnel allowed nurses to extend the reach of physicians in areas not conducive to rapid travel. FNS publicity materials emphasized: "No other plan would be feasible in a country where the difficulties of transportation are so acute."[28] Moreover, according to Breckinridge:

> In a service designed, like ours, for a remotely rural area, the hospital and medical director are like the palm of a hand from which fingers radiate in several directions. It is possible, under this system, for a hardy physician to be responsible for the medical needs of some nine thousand people annually, many of whom he does not meet, whereas he could serve little more than a five-mile radius without his nurse–midwives.[29]

When she determined the locations of district nursing centers and the confines of each district nurse's territory, Breckinridge ignored county lines and other artificial delineations. Instead, Frontier Nursing Service districts "followed the waterways, the natural arteries of travel and trade."[30]

Moreover, Breckinridge invested the additional time and money necessary to guard against the effects of natural disasters that were all too common in the remotely rural, mountainous area. Breckinridge insisted that foundations of all FNS buildings reached solid rock for long-term stability and that "every building, down to the barns and chicken houses, must be located well above the highest floodwater mark." After conferring with local people experienced in the perils of the geography, Breckinridge also resisted the temptation to build on easily accessible, flat, bottom land. Through construction choices, Breckinridge ensured that FNS buildings were safe.[31]

Because frontier nurses traveled by horseback daily between remote mountain cabins and district nursing centers, they devised an efficient system to carry critical supplies. Specially designed, extra-roomy saddlebags fit the bill. Fashioned by hand by a man from a nearby county, frontier saddlebags were large enough to fit a long list of necessary supplies and were made of soft, high–quality leather to enhance durability and comfort for both horse and rider. Furthermore, the saddlebags bore special metal buttons on which nurses fastened a washable lining. One saddlebag with white lining was for midwifery equipment, and the other, lined with blue checked fabric, served general nursing needs. The nurses took special care in packing to evenly distribute the 42 pounds of equipment and to protect valuable and delicate supplies.[32] For further protection of supplies in the saddlebags, riding instructors taught new frontier nurses how to control a horse in a distinct manner called a "running walk." This type of gait caused the rider to sway from side to side but prevented breakage of precious medication ampules, an all-too-common occurrence if a horse trotted. Because the horses had an uncanny ability to know when they were headed home, it was crucial that the nurses learned how to prevent the horses from galloping in their quest to hasten the homeward journey. Controlling the horses in such instances saved medications.[33]

Thus, much public health nursing and midwifery care needed to be done when Breckinridge identified Eastern Kentucky as an ideal location to demonstrate that a group of educated and energetic nurses could make sweeping changes in the health of rural people.

CHALLENGES OF A RURAL NURSE–MIDWIFERY SERVICE

Frontier nurse–midwives faced daunting difficulties in reaching their patients, including an inaccessible and scanty road network, treacherous terrain, and extreme mountain weather. Between the service's inception in 1925 and the early 1950s, nurses traversed the miles between patients and from hospital to clinics almost exclusively by horse on trails crisscrossing the steep, thickly forested mountainsides. Not only were motorized vehicles unaffordable to the fledgling and cash-poor service, according to Breckinridge: "There wasn't a motor road within sixty miles when our work began . . ."[34] Extreme weather and treacherous terrain created additional difficulties for frontier nurses that nurses in other settings could only imagine. One of the most dangerous seasons for the nurses was early spring, in which heavy rains and rushing streams and rivers created temporary obstacles to reaching the patients. Breckinridge reported the effects of a series of December rainstorms that left the service to cope with "inundated roads, heaps of mire and quicksand, great washouts and gullies." Even worse was the fact that the district nursing centers were "marooned from one another by a waste of angry waters tearing madly down the craggy slopes into the creeks and branches and bearing with them to the river logs and boulders and the earth itself in landslides." However, with her characteristic understatement and a demonstration of the hardiness and positive attitude necessary for frontier nurses, Breckinridge concluded that such devastation was "a bit disheartening." Moreover, obstacles did not keep frontier nurses from caring for their patients: "Meanwhile [the midwives] crossed precarious swinging bridges and climbed mountains on all fours to catch five babies who made their advent during the storms and floods."[35]

Breckinridge faced another serious challenge related to the remote and rural environment: finding physicians to provide consultations on complicated cases. Few doctors were willing to live and work in such a remote area, away from patients who could pay for a physician's care and away from the technological medical advances to which physicians were accustomed. Scott Breckinridge, Mary Breckinridge's cousin and prominent

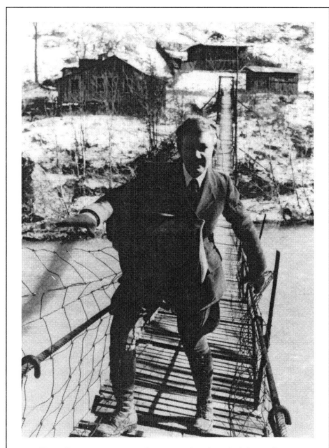

*Frontier nurse crossing a swinging bridge above
a rushing river.*

● ● ● ● ●

Lexington physician, made the point in a letter to the editor of the Lexington newspaper:

> The raising of the standards of medical education and the increasing need of laboratory and hospital facilities for the satisfactory practice of medicine creates difficulties persuading qualified practitioners to locate in isolated communities where those facilities are lacking and where the returns for the services rendered are, at best, most meager.[36]

In fact, there were often periods in which frontier nurses cared for their patients without the benefit of either a medical director or local physicians whom the nurses could summon quickly in an emergency.[37]

Often the nurses relied solely on written *Medical Routines* to handle problems and then consulted with the physician long after the situation had resolved.[38] Breckinridge reported in her autobiography that a frontier nurse-midwife often was not only required to "hold the fort until the Medical Director can reach her, but she often has to take the final responsibility in the knowledge that he cannot reach her in time." This was true when the nurses faced an especially dangerous and time-sensitive obstetric complication, postpartum hemorrhage. During the early years of the service, the experience and intuition of a frontier nurse foretold difficulties with a particular birth of a woman in her mountain cabin. As the nurse predicted, trouble began when the woman began to bleed dangerously after the baby was born but before the placenta was delivered. The nurse acted rapidly and in accordance with her training and the service's *Medical Routines*. She "slipped on a fresh glove and went up into the uterus after the placenta. She acted so quickly, and the patient responded afterward to restoratives so well, that the mother, who would have died before the doctor could reach her, made an uneventful recovery.[39]

At other times, patients needing surgery could wait until non-FNS physician specialists held occasional clinics in the FNS area. This 1941 clinic, described in FNS publicity materials, was typical:

> With Dr. F. W. Urton as operator and Dr. D. M. Dollar as anesthetist we had our tonsil clinic again this year from October 19 through the 21. These two distinguished men gave all of this time out of their busy lives to meet the really desperate needs of our children whose bad tonsils would otherwise mean sickness, hearing disabilities and other complications, not only through the winter months but for life.[40]

At other times nurses referred patients to physicians in cities hundreds of miles away from the patients' homes, necessitating difficult travel out of the mountains. Affiliations with children's hospitals in Louisville and

Cincinnati and with surgeons in Lexington helped meet the needs of injured and ill children who needed care that was unavailable in the mountains.[41] Breckinridge described the care of one such child, a 4-year-old boy who had been badly burned the year before: "His right arm had grown to his side like a wing." After miles of travel over mountain trails to a railroad and then a train ride to Lexington, the doctor released the small, imprisoned arm and "grafted skin over the ruined tissues."[42]

Breckinridge and other FNS leaders also faced the challenge of recruiting and retaining staff members who were highly skilled *and* were willing to tolerate a rustic standard of living. Breckinridge and her staff did not want to attract just *any* nurse. Based on his interviews with Breckinridge, Ernest Poole praised frontier nurses in his 1932 book, *Nurses on Horseback*, by saying that the nurses primarily relied on their own skills: "The nurses are so often thrown on their own resources, in matters even of life and death, in the mountain cabins, that none but the ablest women carefully trained are adequate."[43]

Moreover, successful frontier nurses were hardy and altruistic, and possessed a pioneering spirit. Writing in a 1940 *American Journal of Nursing* article, FNS Assistant Director Dorothy Buck described the type of nurses she sought:

> The Frontier Nursing Service would not appeal to all nurses. Those looking for high salaries; those who find their pleasure only in concerts, plays, picture galleries—those should not seek happiness in the Frontier Nursing Service. But to those who prefer the silent woodland path to the crowded city pavements, to those who enjoy the friendship of dogs and horses—to those we offer a land of dreams come true.[44]

ADVANTAGES OF THE RURAL SETTING

In spite of difficulties, the frontier's remote surroundings also provided benefits. The rural setting allowed Breckinridge to craft a particular image of the service to enhance fundraising and staff recruiting efforts.[45] To her wealthy, urban-dwelling friends, she emphasized that FNS patients, mostly of Scottish descent, were the rural, worthy poor, hard-working, and proud. A visiting journalist noted that, despite "desperate" poverty, "whole families work early and late, plowing, planting, building fences, cutting wood, tending gardens, cows, chickens, and mules." Mary Breckinridge reinforced the concept for the journalist: "They're too proud to beg. In all the years of our service I could count on the fingers of my two hands all those who have asked us for charity."[46]

In her autobiography, *Wide Neighborhoods*, Breckinridge framed the Kentucky mountaineer's "isolation from modern times" in a positive light.

She argued that this isolation encouraged Kentuckians to retain a "code of honor long after it had been abandoned by the outside world."[47] A key feature of this code was chivalry to women. Not only would this appeal to potential donors who longed for a simpler, bygone era, but this ideal enhanced recruiting potential for nurses and college-age FNS volunteers called couriers. Breckinridge wrote: "Our nurses go out on calls with any man, anywhere, at any hour of any night, if he comes for them. Our young couriers can ride alone over the most remote trails with a safety that would not be theirs in some parts of our great cities."[48]

Breckinridge went on to emphasize that the mountain people—people from rural backgrounds—were worth saving: "Fully 80% of the men who direct our great corporations came from rural regions."[49] Breckinridge argued that robust growth of the nation depended on caring for rural children. She continued by saying, "Mother Nature has a way of reaching over rich nurseries to her own rough bosom and picking great men from the soil. So let us give such boys a chance. Help mothers to have their children well born."[50]

Breckinridge relied on imagery of the worthy poor to accomplish her mission of raising funds to support the work of the FNS. Indeed, the $5 fee that the FNS charged patients throughout the 1920s, 1930s, and 1940s for complete midwifery care, attendance at the birth, and multiple nursing visits after the birth was woefully inadequate to finance the organization's work.[51] Thus, Breckinridge's fundraising strategy relied on the development and cultivation of volunteer committees in the Northeast and Midwest, composed of well-to-do and influential citizens in cities such as Washington, DC, New York, Chicago, and Boston. Committee members included such prominent individuals as Clara Ford, wife of Henry Ford.[52]

Breckinridge used a romanticized version of the FNS's rural environment to allow FNS committee members and potential donors to vicariously return to an idyllic era. In fact, Breckinridge referred to her trips between remote eastern Kentucky and the large cities when she attended the committee meetings as travel "in and out of centuries . . . Each time I made the trip I moved from the nineteenth into the twentieth century, and back from the twentieth into the nineteenth."[53] Skillful use of the service's *Quarterly Bulletin*, a publication that FNS leaders sent to donors and friends of the service, allowed Breckinridge to create a particular image of the nurses' work and the setting in which they accomplished it. *Quarterly Bulletin* articles incorporated images of remote terrain, overlaid with visions of great beauty, allowing readers (and potential donors) to return to a bygone era when life was simple and appealingly rugged. Breckinridge included this description of the rugged beauty on her district rounds on horseback:

> We first rode up "Hell-for-certain"—a horribly rough creek about eight miles long. Then we got into a great primeval forest extending for many miles in all directions, with trails leading in a most confusing zigzag.

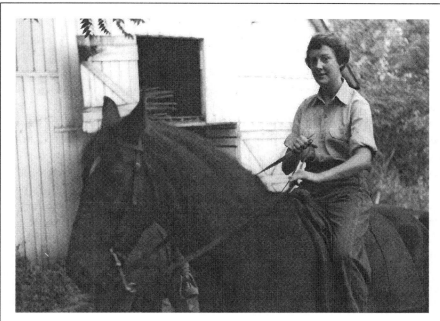

Frontier district nurse.

● ● ● ● ●

But you could comb the world without finding anything more beautiful than that forest. No lover of luxury would ever see that beauty because he wouldn't be able to reach it. It can only be reached by horseback riders, and hard riders at that.[54]

Breckinridge continued in the same article by describing a district nursing center:

The center at Red Bird is perfectly exquisite—a rambling log building with a big veranda, a living room with an open stone fire, two bedrooms for the nurses, a large waiting room for the patients. The barn has stalls for visiting horses, a good saddle room, a feed room screened against rats, and the whole structure is of solid oak. The whole property is the gift of Mrs. Henry Ford.[55]

Breckinridge concluded by saying, "I give this in detail so that you can visualize one center."[56] Doubtless, she hoped that wealthy friends of the FNS would visualize it so well that they would send the funds to build another center.

Another facet of Frontier's fundraising plan involved the use of couriers, the college-aged daughters and nieces of FNS donors and committee members. Couriers traveled to the FNS and stayed for 6 or 8 weeks, volunteering their time to care for horses, ferry messages and supplies, escort visitors around the FNS territory, assist nurses, and generally do anything that needed to be done. Couriers' work benefited the FNS by providing thousands of hours of unpaid work each year.[57]

That former couriers became lifelong advocates for Frontier was an even more far-reaching benefit of the courier program. Indeed, couriers took the FNS message out of the mountains and strengthened long lasting ties between donors and the FNS. Couriers believed they were an essential part of a vital mission. One former courier credited Frontier with "an ability to make you feel that you were a very important cog in their machine more quickly than anything else I've ever become involved in."[58] Seeing the service's work up close allowed the couriers to return home as effective ambassadors for the Frontier Nursing Service and to tell their friends and family members of the incredible work being done in Kentucky. In her journal, one courier named Susan described a home visit she made with one of the nurses on horseback. Susan was amazed at the dozens of people the nurse spoke to on their rounds, asking about their health or the health of some member of their family. The courier remarked: "This trip makes me see what the whole organization is about—why the nurses have to go by horseback and how the people really need them." Similarly, Susan delighted in watching a nurse skillfully attend a laboring woman in a mountain cabin. She recorded in her journal: "Around five minutes of twelve the baby was born without too much trouble . . . It was a boy and eight pounds worth. I've never seen anyone work as gently or as deftly."[59]

The rural and rustic setting also appealed to nurses. FNS nurses often sought the adventure of being a famed and romantic "nurse on horseback," in a lovely, natural mountain setting. To entice nurses to work in the Frontier Nursing Service and students to attend Frontier's graduate school of midwifery, Breckinridge wrote numerous articles for her target audience of young, public health-focused nurses in the *American Journal of Nursing* and women's magazines. Prospective nurses were also enthralled with the poignant and colorful tales of the Frontier midwives working in the Kentucky mountains in journalist Ernest Poole's 1932 book, *Nurses on Horseback*. Stories like this one—full of drama and several exciting and healthy births—were doubtless instrumental in luring nurses to the FNS.

One nurse wrote in a routine report about her ultimately successful quest to arrive at a mountain cabin in time for the birth of a baby, in spite of multiple flood-swollen waterways in her path:

A big flood Friday and Saturday smashed everything along the river. At nine o'clock on Friday night, a man came for me from Wolf Creek. He had to swim down the road, and we couldn't get back the way he came, so we went up Hurricane Creek on the most terrible trail. We had to swim Coon Creek four times, and he waded up to his neck nine times. Reached his cabin at midnight, delivered the baby early next morning.[60]

Safely back at her clinic home, the weary nurse prepared for a well-deserved rest until another urgent call came. With the rainwater continuing to choke the area's waterways, the beleaguered nurse was forced to abandon her horse and travel by boat this time: "The river was so swift, the boat skimmed past the landing like a piece of driftwood. Landed safely below the ford in the M.'s bottom field, and reached the cabin that night. At two a.m. I caught an eleven-pound boy."[61]

In fact, even as Jeeps began to replace horses, frontier nurses often took the perils of terrain and weather in stride. In fact, the nurses even found humor in the hazardous conditions in which they worked and drove. In a *Quarterly Bulletin*, under a headline of "Understatement of the Week," this incident illustrates FNS nurses' mettle and their senses of humor:

During a spell of icy weather two of our district nurses were riding in their Jeep along a narrow road, when the Jeep went into a skid and turned over the bank and slid into the icy waters of the creek. One nurse decided it was not time for her to drown and scrambled on to the bank. She turned to look for her companion. To her surprise she found her sitting on the Jeep which was lying on its side in the creek, and remarking to a neighbor man who had rushed to their assistance: "Oh, we were on our way to see your baby. We will be there in a little while!"[62]

LIVING AND WORKING IN IMPOVERISHED MOUNTAIN COMMUNITIES

FNS nurses carefully negotiated the intricacies of living and working in remote Appalachian communities. Extreme poverty was an important factor in bringing the FNS to the area and, despite nearly a decade of gains in improving their health, Mary Breckinridge pronounced in the early 1930s that "We've still to attack their poverty."[63] Later, Breckinridge wrote:

Not even in the war-devastated areas of northern France have I known greater poverty than we had in the Kentucky mountains in our early days, at a time when living conditions beyond the mountains were good. It just wasn't possible for a man to raise enough to feed his family on steep land, utterly unsuited for any kind of a crop but timber. . .[64]

This poverty deeply affected FNS nurses, including a midwifery student who recalled: "I was a different kind of person after working in Kentucky.

It was a rude awakening that these types of conditions existed in my own country. I gained a deeper understanding of the effects of poverty in America."[65] Poverty also affected families' abilities to adhere to middle-class norms of hygiene and health standards. Another midwifery student recalled that, due to concerns about acquiring intestinal parasites and bacteria, FNS staff never drank the water when visiting a patient's mountain cabin because most families "didn't have access to proper sanitation."[66]

Despite the abject poverty in which many of the patients lived, mountain culture dictated that hospitality should supersede all and FNS nurses benefited from it. After an FNS nurse attended a birth in a mountain cabin, she sat down to a hearty meal prepared for the occasion. One nurse fondly recalled delicious meals of "fried eggs, oatmeal, cornbread, berry jam, and milk that they had prepared for us."[67] Some nurses, like this one, valued the

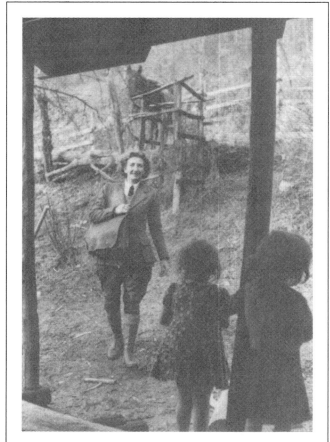

Frontier nurse visiting mountain family.

● ● ● ● ●

meaning of this celebratory meal, in spite of any health risks it might impart: "We soon learned not to refuse anything they offered us to eat, as they were very sensitive to any seeming lack of appreciation of their offering to share what little they had."[68]

USING THE FULL EXTENT OF KNOWLEDGE

In some ways, nurses also benefited from the lack of physicians in the area. That nurses were willing to sequester themselves in a remote and rural area in which physicians did not want to work served to minimize physicians' concerns of competition with the newly established profession of nurse-midwifery. As a group, physicians were satisfied with allowing FNS nurses to practice there.

Physicians' absence provided tangible benefits for the service's Frontier Graduate School of Midwifery (FGSM), a training program founded in 1939 that supplied the FNS with a steady stream of staff.[69] Far away from any established center of physician education, FGSM students did not need to compete with physicians-in-training for clinical experiences. School alumni found the relative lack of physicians in southeastern Kentucky, particularly the lack of medical students, a *plus* for their midwifery training there. Attending the births of twins and breech babies was something that would not have happened had the students chosen another school such as the Lobenstine midwifery school in urban New York City. There, readily available physicians-in-training would have taken these exciting training experiences, leaving midwifery students without the opportunities to develop these skills.[70]

The advanced training in difficult skills, coupled with the remote environment, proved to be a fortuitous match for many students at Frontier's school who planned to serve in missionary roles in developing countries around the world. One graduate later wrote her old friends at Frontier:

> I have been to Haiti and back. The country is beautiful. . . . so many things reminded me of the Kentucky hills. The roads are rough, steep and narrow with creeks and rivers to ford. At the particular mission compound I visited they needed a clinic built, and a nurse to ride a burro to reach the people up in the mountains—that is *just the training I have had at Frontier*, so they want me to return.[71]

CONCLUSION

Beginning in 1925 nurses working for the Frontier Nursing Service provided care to the citizens living in remote and rural eastern Kentucky, a mountainous area in which few physicians wanted to live and practice. There, FNS nurses overcame significant geographic and economic challenges to provide access to care to many with dire health needs. Nurses negotiated unique cultural situations to live and work in meaningful ways with members of the mountain communities. The rural setting also permitted certain advantages. Images of the appealingly rustic setting enhanced private fundraising efforts through imagery of a bygone era and romantic versions of nurses on horseback. Moreover, frontier nurses and graduate students enjoyed minimal competition with physicians for the rights to practice in the remote and underserved area. Together, the setting and its needs challenged the FNS nurses to use the full extent of their knowledge and skill to meet patients' needs.

NOTES

1. Mary Breckinridge, *Wide Neighborhoods* (Lexington, KY: The University Press of Kentucky, 1952), 228. Emphasis with italicized words the same as in the original text.

2. James C. Klotter, *The Breckinridges of Kentucky* (Lexington, KY: The University Press of Kentucky, 2006).

3. Mary Breckinridge's life has been well documented by many historians and biographers. See Carol Crowe-Carraco, "Mary Breckinridge and the Frontier Nursing Service," *Register of the Kentucky Historical Society* 76 (July 1978): 179–91; Nancy Schrom Dye, "Mary Breckinridge, the Frontier Nursing Service and the Introduction of Nurse-Midwifery in the United States," *Bulletin of the History of Medicine* 57 (1983): 485–507; and Melanie Beals Goan, *Mary Breckinridge: The Frontier Nursing Service and Rural Health in Appalachia* (Chapel Hill, NC: The University of North Carolina Press, 2008). See also Helen Deiss Irvin, *Women in Kentucky* (Lexington, KY: University Press of Kentucky, 1979), 116–18. For additional reading about the Frontier Nursing Service in general, see Marie Bartlett, *The Frontier Nursing Service: America's First Rural Nurse-Midwife Service and School* (Jefferson, NC: McFarland, 2008).

4. Mary Breckinridge worked through some of her profound grief over the loss of her beloved son, Breckinridge ("Breckie") Thompson by writing a slim volume: Mary Breckinridge Thompson, *Breckie, His Four Years, 1914–1918* (New York, NY: Privately published, 1918).

5. Breckinridge, *Wide Neighborhoods*, 75. For additional reading about the U.S. Children's Bureau, see Kriste Lindenmeyer, *A Right to Childhood: The U.S. Children's Bureau and Child Welfare, 1912–1946* (Chicago, IL: University of Illinois Press, 1997).

6. Goan, *Mary Breckinridge*, 53. For additional reading about Mary Breckinridge's service to CARD, see Anne G. Campbell, "Mary Breckinridge and the American Committee for Devastated France: The Foundations of the Frontier Nursing Service," *Register of the Kentucky Historical Society* 82 (Summer 1984): 257–76.

7. For additional reading about Progressive Era work to decrease infant mortality, see Solomon Newmayer, "The Warfare against Infant Mortality," *Annals of the*

American Academy of Political and Social Science 37 (1911): 532–42; and Richard Arthur Bolt, "Fundamental Factors in Infant Mortality," *Annals of the American Academy of Political and Social Science* 48 (1921): 9–16.

8. Breckinridge, *Wide Neighborhoods*, 111.

9. Breckinridge, *Wide Neighborhoods*, 111.

10. Breckinridge, *Wide Neighborhoods*, 158.

11. Quoted in Breckinridge, *Wide Neighborhoods*, 158–159.

12. Breckinridge, *Wide Neighborhoods*, 158.

13. Laura Ettinger, *Nurse-Midwifery: The Birth of a New American Profession* (Columbus, OH: The Ohio State University Press, 2006), 36.

14. Breckinridge, *Wide Neighborhoods*, 229.

15. Breckinridge, *Wide Neighborhoods*, 116.

16. Breckinridge, *Wide Neighborhoods*, 116.

17. Crowe-Carraco, "Mary Breckinridge and the Frontier Nursing Service," 181.

18. Goan, *Mary Breckinridge*, 83. See also Mary Breckinridge, "An Adventure in Midwifery: The Nurse-on-Horseback Gets a 'Soon Start'," reprint from *Survey Graphic* (October 1926), American College of Nurse-Midwives Collection, National Library of Medicine, MS C 330a, box 63, folder 41.

19. Goan, *Mary Breckinridge*, 85.

20. Breckinridge, *Wide Neighborhoods*, 160.

21. Goan, *Mary Breckinridge*, 87.

22. For the viewpoint of a public health nurse (non-midwife) who traveled to Kentucky to explore the possibility of working there, see Winifred Rand, "Impressions of a Public Health Nursing Service in the Kentucky Mountains," *American Journal of Nursing* 29 (May 1929): 527–30.

23. For an overview of the medical needs from the viewpoint of a physician, the FNS medical director, see John H. Kooser, "Mountain Medicine," reprint from the *Journal of Medicine* (April 1934), Frontier Nursing Service Collection (hereafter FNSC) University of Kentucky Libraries (hereafter UKL) 85M1, box 35, folder 14.

24. Ernest Poole, *Nurses on Horseback*, (New York: The Macmillan Company, 1932), 38. For vivid stories about the exigencies of life in mountainous Eastern Kentucky in the 1930s written for a lay audience, see Caroline Gardner, *Clever Country: Kentucky Mountain Trails* (New York, NY: Fleming H. Revell, 1931). See also Anna May January, "Friday at Frontier Nursing Service," *Public Health Nursing* 40 (December 1948): 601–602.

25. Breckinridge, *Wide Neighborhoods*, 190.

26. Breckinridge, *Wide Neighborhoods*, 190.

27. Breckinridge, *Wide Neighborhoods*, 244–45.

28. Frontier Nursing Service "Organization and Supervision of Field Work of the Frontier Nursing Service," reprint from the *Quarterly Bulletin of the Frontier Nursing Service, Inc* 10 (Winter 1935): 3.

29. Breckinridge, *Wide Neighborhoods*, 229.

30. Breckinridge, *Wide Neighborhoods*, 229.

31. Breckinridge, *Wide Neighborhoods*, 230.

32. Delivery Bag Equipment, circa 1940s. FNSC UKL 2005 MS47, box 228; Breckinridge, *Wide Neighborhoods*, 176; and Vanda Summers, "Saddle-Bag and Log Cabin Technique," reprinted from the *Quarterly Bulletin of the Frontier Nursing Service, Inc.*

33. Maria Mariscal, interviewed by Marie C. Wright, FNU Collection.

34. Breckinridge, *Wide Neighborhoods*, 167.

35. Breckinridge, *Wide Neighborhoods*, 196.

36. Scott Breckinridge, Letter to the Editor of the *Lexington Herald*, July 24, 1931, FNSC UKL 85M1, box 344, folder 2.

37. Frontier leaders faced particular difficulties in keeping a medical director during the 1940s and 1950s. After Dr. John Kooser, Medical Director for 12 years, left FNS to join the Navy in support of the war effort in 1943, subsequent medical directors remained only for periods of a few months or a few years. At other times, there was no medical director. See Nancy Dammann, *A Social History of the Frontier Nursing Service* (Sun City, AZ: Social Change Press, 1982), 87.

38. For more about FNS Medical Routines concerning medications, see Arlene W. Keeling, *Nursing and the Privilege of Prescription, 1893–2000* (Columbus, OH: The Ohio State University Press, 2007).

39. Breckinridge, *Wide Neighborhoods*, 308.

40. "Field Notes," *QB 17*, 2 (Autumn 1941): 68–69.

41. FNS publicity brochure: "Frontier Nursing Service in War" (April 1943), p. 3, Berea College Special Collections.

42. Breckinridge, *Wide Neighborhoods*, 256.

43. Poole, *Nurses on Horseback*, 31.

44. Buck, "The Nurses on Horseback Ride On," 994–95.

45. Historian Laura Ettinger makes similar points in the FNS chapter of her excellent study of midwifery, *Nurse-Midwifery: The Birth of a New American Profession* (Columbus, OH: The Ohio State University Press, 2006).

46. Ernest Poole, "The Nurse on Horseback Has Brought New Life and Hope to the Kentucky Mountaineers," *Good Housekeeping* (June 1932), page numbers unavailable.

47. Breckinridge, *Wide Neighborhoods*, 170.

48. Breckinridge, *Wide Neighborhoods*, 170.

49. Poole, "The Nurse on Horseback," page number unavailable.

50. Poole, "The Nurse on Horseback."

51. Edith Reeves Solenberger, "Nurses on Horseback," *Hygeia: The Health Magazine Published by the American Medical Association* (July 1931), p. 635. FNSC UKL 85M1, box 35, folder 6.

52. Goan, *Mary Breckinridge*, 111.

53. Breckinridge, *Wide Neighborhoods*, 194.

54. "Rounds," *QB* 5, 2 (September 1929): 5–6.

55. *QB* 5, 2 (September 1929): 6.

56. *QB* 5, 2 (September 1929): 6.

57. For additional reading about Frontier's courier program, see Anne Z. Cockerham, *Unbridled Service: Growing Up and Giving Back as a Frontier Courier, 1928–2010* (Louisville, KY: Butler Books, 2014 in press).

58. Interview with Mardi Perry, FNS Oral History Project, 1979OH146 FNSC 053, Louie B. Nunn Center for Oral History, UKL, p. 29 of transcript.

59. Diary of Susan Spencer, September 20, 1948, FNSC, UKL, 2005MS47, box 40, folder 3.

60. Poole, *Nurses on Horseback*, 32–33.

61. Poole, *Nurses on Horseback*, 33.

62. *QB* 37, 3 (Winter 1961): 43.

63. Mary Breckinridge, writing in *Good Housekeeping* in the early 1930s, quoted in Goan, *Mary Breckinridge*: 146.

64. Breckinridge, *Wide Neighborhoods*, 266.

65. Gwen Buchanan, interviewed by Paulomi Niles, FNU Collection.

66. Virginia Bowling, interviewed by Christina S. Scribner, FNU Collection.

67. Elizabeth Walton, letter to unspecified recipient, May 28, 1945, FNU Collection.

68. Elizabeth Walton, email to Denise Barrett, December 15, 2006, FNU Collection.

69. For additional reading about Frontier's nurse-midwifery training program, see Anne Z. Cockerham and Arlene W. Keeling, *Rooted in the Mountains, Reaching to the World: Stories of Nursing and Midwifery at Kentucky's Frontier School, 1939–1989* (Louisville, KY: Butler Books, 2012).

70. Madonna Spratt, interviewed by Michele Cohen, FNU Collection.

71. *QB* 37, 4 (Spring 1961): 25. Emphasis added.

7

•••••

Migrant Nursing in the Great Depression: Floods, Flies, and the Farm Security Administration

•••••

ARLENE W. KEELING

One family . . . lived in a shelter built against a wire fence. Two bed sheets formed the roof, and old quilts and burlap made the sidewalls. In it lived six people. The baby lay on the bed, covered completely with a quilt to protect it from the flies; a little living skeleton with a rodent expression produced from sunken eyes and two protruding teeth and wracked with whooping cough. An undersized eleven-year- old answered questions, as both parents were picking cotton for dear life. "The baby don't get milk," she told me bluntly "he gits [sic] what we git [sic]: soup."[1]

IN 1941, GOVERNMENT NURSE MARY SEARS wrote of her experience nursing migratory farmworkers and their families in California during the Great Depression. Her work was part of President Franklin D. Roosevelt's New Deal "migrant medical care program"—a program under the Agricultural Workers Health and Medical Association (AWHMA) established by the Farm Security Administration (FSA) in 1938. At its peak, its services extended to over "a million people."[2] Nurses were key players in the program, employed first by the state and later by the AWHMA to keep the migrants healthy, keep them from spreading disease, and keep them working in the fields.

THE GREAT DEPRESSION AND THE DUST BOWL

With the stock market crash in 1929, millions of Americans lost their jobs; within a few short years, manufacturing "all but ground to a halt . . . the automobile industry was operating at 20 percent of capacity, and the steel industry at just 12 percent."[3] Rural areas were particularly devastated—farm income plummeted from $6.7 billion in 1929 to $2.3 billion over the course of 3 years. At the same time, tractors were replacing manual labor. When a devastating drought hit the Midwest in 1933, crops would not grow at all. As author Timothy Egan noted, it was the "worst hard time."[4] Soon farmers, devastated by drought, dust, and dropping crop prices, could not cover their expenses.[5] Small farmers lost their property to foreclosure; workers and sharecroppers, replaced by new farm machinery, were "tractored off" the land.

Many of these destitute families migrated from the great American Dust Bowl states to California in search of work. The majority of the poverty-stricken farm families did not leave their homes willingly. Rather, they left their homes to save themselves and their children from starvation, following

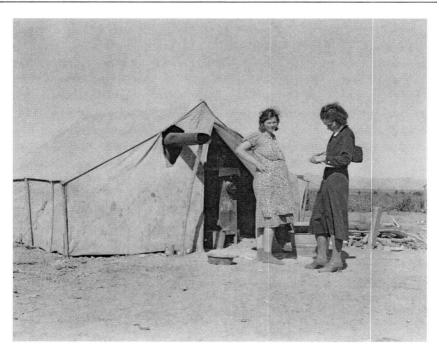

Public health nurse making prenatal visit, Imperial Valley, California.

● ● ● ● ●

Route 66 in their battered jalopies; the cars crammed with their belongings and their dirty, barefooted children.

On arrival in California, some of the migrants settled in and around towns throughout the state, joining family members already living there, but thousands converged in the San Joaquin and Imperial Valleys and became migratory farm laborers. The migrants followed the crop harvest from season to season, picking citrus, lettuce, and walnuts near San Fernando; potatoes, grapes, and cotton near Shafter; onions at Arvin; and then heading north to the Yuba City area to harvest grapes, peaches, and apricots. Everywhere they went the migrant workers drove down wages by their sheer numbers and willing-ness to work for less than $1.00 a day.[6] Stereotyped by mainstream California residents as "Okies" or "Arkies," the newcomers would serve as a major labor force for harvesting fruits, vegetables, and cotton. These predominantly White Americans would also displace Mexican, Japanese, and Chinese laborers who had traditionally worked in agriculture in California.

The living conditions that Mary Sears described were not unique. According to U.S. President Franklin D. Roosevelt, one third of U.S. citizens were "ill-housed, ill-clad, and ill-nourished" during the Great Depression of the 1930s.[7] Chief among these were the almost 200,000 migrant farm families from Oklahoma, Arkansas, and Missouri who ended up on the nation's west coast, "concentrated in appalling numbers, led by the faint hope of a new life and fabulous tales of work to be found in cotton fields, orange groves, and grape vineyards."[8]

THE DITCH CAMPS

Homeless, the migrants lived in camps owned by their employers or in make-shift squatter camps that sprung up haphazardly along irrigation ditches close to the fields and orchards.[9] A report, published by the California State Relief Administration in 1936, noted that families congregated in the ditch bank camps "without public supervision or regulation."[10] Conditions in these camps were abysmal. According to the state's report: "Old tents, gun-nysacks, dry-good boxes and scrap tin. These are the materials from which the dwellings are constructed . . . The shacks are without floors . . . very dirty and swarming with clouds of flies."[11]

Some families did not even have shacks and slept on the ground, storing their blankets in their dilapidated cars during the daytime. The children were "dressed in rags, their hair encrusted with dirt, complexions pasty white. . . ."[12] Despite their poverty, the destitute migrant workers and their families did not qualify for California state relief; most counties required that individuals were eligible for relief only after they had established permanent residency for 1 to 3 years.[13] Local citizens soon turned against the homeless itinerants, closing doors that would access medical care, education, and housing.

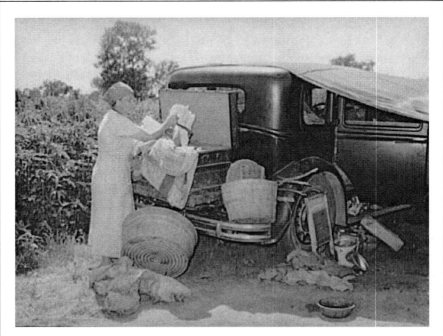

Living out of the car.

♦ ♦ ♦ ♦ ♦

Fear of the spread of disease was one cause for the rising prejudice against the disheveled newcomers and their "grimy, coughing children."[14] Given the conditions in the camps, that fear was well founded. There was never enough water in the camps and only the rare outhouse. Sometimes the only source of water was the irrigation ditch—half-filled with muddy water and used for a toilet in addition to washing, cooking, and bathing.[15] Sometimes drinking water was brought in from a distant ice plant.[16] Under these conditions, the camps became breeding grounds for contagious disease. Outbreaks of typhoid and smallpox were common; tuberculosis, dysentery, and diarrhea were endemic.[17] Other commonly occurring diseases were conjunctivitis, scarlet fever, gastrointestinal diseases (particularly in infants), and upper respiratory infections, especially in the winter months. Some diseases were much more serious. As public health nurse Mary Sears recalled, "Polio was one of the horrors."[18]

PROMOTING HEALTH

Terrified of epidemics spreading throughout California, and faced with the problem of providing the migrants with the basic necessities of food, clothing, and shelter, the California State Emergency Relief Administration (SERA) built several farm labor camps using federal and state funds.[19] Something also had to be done about the migrants' medical needs, however, and on November 14, 1937, the California Medical Association went on record as favoring a statewide program of health insurance to provide "low-cost medical care for thousands of migrants who could not pay standard fees for medical, dental, and hospital services."[20] Local county physicians, paid on a fee-for-service basis, would serve these camps, along with a few county public health nurses. The nurse, paid by the AWHMA and State Health Department, would have a great deal of autonomy, practicing "rather freelance in her territory, using her own judgment in planning work."[21]

State leaders then asked Ralph C. Williams, MD, the FSA's Chief Medical officer in Washington, to come to California to "help work out a medical aid program."[22] Thus, in January 1938, Williams accompanied State Department of Health George Uhl, MD, on a trip through California's San Joaquin and Imperial Valleys, documenting the scope of the problems.[23]

The problems extended throughout the entire state. Malnutrition plagued the migrants, despite the fact that they worked picking vegetables and fruits for their employers. Destitute, most of the migrants managed to survive on a diet of hotcakes made from flour, salt, and water; salt pork, boiled beans, and occasionally corn bread and molasses or baking powder biscuits with gravy.[24] Health problems followed. According to one report, a family of eight had been subsisting for over 2 weeks on hotcakes made of "flour, salt and water" and cooked in grease from the fat of a salt pork rind the mother had managed to save. The mother then presented to the nurse, having noticed "the skin of her hands and wrists cracking and becoming infected . . . her gums sore and bleeding."[25]

Sometimes the children had nothing to eat; at other times, during "potato-picking season" they might have "potato sandwiches for lunch—sliced raw potato between two slices of bread."[26] According to Williams, "most every child in camp" suffered from "nutritional defects."[27] Many had pellagra, a preventable disease caused by lack of niacin.[28] In California, among migrant children alone, nutritional defects were 34% of all defects in 1936 to 1937, and 38% in 1937 to 1938.[29] As one public health nurse exclaimed: "These people need food, not medicine!"[30]

Stunned by their findings, Williams assigned 18 nutritionists and six United States Public Health (USPHS) nurses to the migrant camps.[31]

By this time the camps numbered almost 13 throughout the state, so the nurses covered more than one.[32] At first, the AWHMA worked with local County Medical Associations to set up panels of physicians in the agricultural areas, establishing a fee schedule with their cooperation. Panels were also made of cooperating dentists, druggists, social workers, and hospitals. In areas of concentrated migrant population, clinics were established "with a nurse, a stenographer clerk, and a part-time physician from the nearest town."

Visiting one camp after another, the local public health nurses made "home visits" to the makeshift shacks, assessing patients' needs and teaching prenatal and well-baby care, hygiene, proper diet, and disease prevention. The lack of proper kitchens, indoor plumbing, refrigeration, and even household goods was a persistent problem. Nurses had to make do with what the family had—teaching young mothers to prepare baby formula using a "saucepan, an empty flask, and a tin spoon"—or how to make a baby bed from an "orange crate and an old quilt."[33] Health teaching was

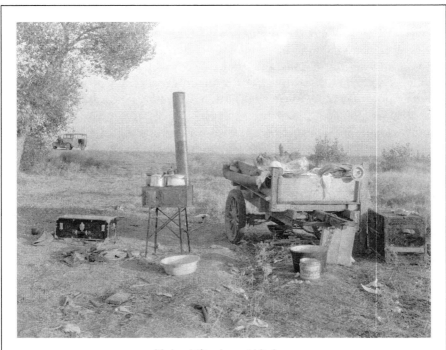

Makeshift migrant kitchen.

● ● ● ● ●

a major aspect of the nurses' role. According to one nurse's report: "One mother had to be made to understand that by bathing four small children with one basin of water using the same towel, she spread impetigo and pink eye among them. It might almost have been better not to have bathed them at all."[34]

Infant, child, and pre- and postnatal care encompassed a large part of the nurse's time, as the migrant mothers were young, inexperienced, and far from relatives who might have helped. In fact, of the 3,376 visits made by two nurses in 1 year, 25% were to infants, 50% to preschool children, 8% to school-age children, and 11% to pre- and postterm mothers. Teaching new mothers how to care for their newborns was particularly important. One nurse's log reflects the extent of the need:

> At the first stop, found my prenatal had turned into a postnatal, not an unusual occurrence, and was in the act of bathing the new baby— dabbling about his head. After a few polite remarks, I asked why she was not tubbing [sic] the baby in this hot weather. 'Well, I ain't never, reckon I might—but no notion as how,' [sic] she replied. This called for a demonstration baby bath, during which time I learned that the baby was bottle fed on a homemade formula . . . The bottle was rinsed before use; when the baby seemed satisfied, the bottle was put to one side for the flies; when the baby cried it was thrust into its mouth. To make a long story short: much education![35]

Because the need for pre- and postnatal teaching was so extensive, the nurses held maternity "conferences" (clinics) in local cabins or "under the trees," spending a week prior to the conference in the camps "building up interest" in attending.[36] Conditions under which the clinics were held were primitive. One clinic was held in the cook house, the "floor of which was dirt." As the nurse recorded: "We had a table, a bench and some lard pails to sit on. . . . With the window open, there was a draught on the babies and with it shut, there was no light. There was no water."[37]

Because the migrants moved so often, following pregnant mothers to provide prenatal and postpartum care was particularly challenging for the nurses. One solution was the use of a "form postal," [postcard] given to each "pre-natal case" so that the mother could send it back to the nurse with her change of address. Even with these postcards, finding the mothers for follow-up visits was not easy, as can be seen in the text on one such card:

> Dear nurse . . . We moved Sunday from Doran's to the Ballard Ranch. Turn south where Hanford road turns north from Corcoran go south

and turn west at first road west, pass one high line then turn north at second high line – about one mile north you can see the camp . . . We are in a tent staked down good with straw in it . . . [38]

Despite their best intentions, the efforts of the local doctors and the few public health nurses working in a demonstration project were simply not enough. Infant mortality was high, as the malnourished mothers could not produce enough milk to breastfeed and they had no money for formula and little knowledge of how to make it if they did. Epidemics raged, and living conditions remained deplorable.[39] Meanwhile, public sentiment against the "Oakies" grew, as the migrants threatened not only jobs, but also the locals' "Americanism, liberties and virtue."[40]

As hordes of dispossessed families continued to pour into the state, things only got worse. The severe floods of 1937 to 1938 brought the situation to a head, as rainy, cold weather combined with poor housing created havoc in the camps. Public Health nurses Edna Rockstroh and Freda Whyte recorded the situation in their annual report:

Very early in the year the heavy rains and storms began their destructive work. Kings County suffered the worst. Much of the cotton, grain and beets were in the old Tulare Lake Basin with the result that, as the basin filled, camp after camp gave way. Levees were built and guarded night and day, but the waters continued their destructive job. There were twelve, at least, of the twenty-three camps visited . . . [that were] evacuated or moved.[41]

The floods changed the nurses' priorities, as demonstrated in a diary entry of March 3, 1938:

On the way out . . . I passed Kopper Camp. The water there was over the bank and creeping up about the tents. I continued on my way, but began to think—after all, what was the use of going on and talking diet and health habits when these conditions were in existence? So again I turned about and drove back to Kopper's. . . . I found all the families congregated in a cabin about ten feet from the highway—no place to go, no money. I drove back to Visalia and contacted the Red Cross. Together the worker from the Red Cross and I made a survey of the conditions of all camps bordering the rivers and creeks and advised the campers that the auditorium in Visalia was to be opened with beds and food for those families whose homes were inundated by flood waters. . . .[42]

News reports of the floods aroused Californians to the growing tragedy. One account described the illnesses that coincided with the floods and the problem of accessing adequate medical care:

> It was the last week in March, the rain kept pouring down and pea pickers kept pouring in, stretching leaking tents over muddy puddles. . . . A week later more than 3,000 people were picking peas . . . scattered over 10 more or less disreputable campsites. At the end of the first week, the nurse had found 151 cases of illness, among them 27 case of whooping cough . . . 23 cases of measles . . . 21 cases of chickenpox . . . and 14 cases of mumps. There were [also] two cases each of trachoma, TB, malaria and pellagra . . . But there was no opportunity for medical care as the Board of Supervisors of that county had voted to hospitalize "extreme emergency cases only."[43]

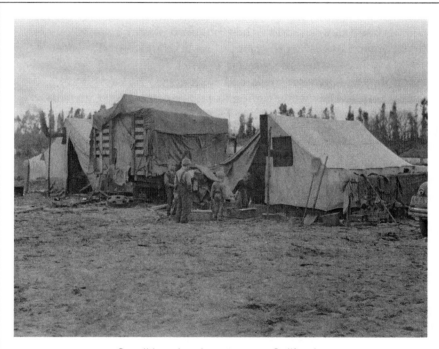

Conditions in migrant camp, California.

● ● ● ● ●

GOVERNMENT "SUITCASE CAMPS"

That spring, the FSA established several more camps, three of which were "entirely and genuinely mobile."[44] These camps had "specially designated trailers and clinics, actually put on wheels. They also had "suitcase shelters" (prefabricated wooden shelters) that could be put up and ready for occupancy within 5 minutes by five men, then loaded onto trucks when the camp was ready to move. In comparison to the squatter camps, the federal ones looked very good. At Arvin, "little well-made box-like houses" replaced the usual tents. An improvement yes, but still cramped and "hellishly hot. . . . Each one just one room for the whole family . . . each with a double bed, an old mattress with bedding on it, pushed under the bed in the daytime."[45] Nonetheless, the mobile camps had "big open spaces" for recreation, a community building for gatherings and dances, and medical and dental trailers in which patients could be seen in clean and dry conditions.

In the mobile camps, as in the standing government camps, the migrants had access to clean water, showers, and laundry facilities. The camps also had supervised day nurseries where children played, napped on cots, and received a noon meal.[46] In the camps, the migrants found respect. According to Mary Sears, when the camp at Brawley first opened, "migrants came pouring in, their jalopies crammed with their worldly goods and their ragged children. They were coming to a place where they were able to wash their rags, sleep off the ground, and live more like human beings."[47] Because they had a chance at fighting the dirt, the flies, and the lack of food, the migrants could return to a semblance of the standard of living previously held before the drought and the economic depression forced them from their homes. At least they could bathe themselves and their children and wash their clothes. They also had access to clean drinking water. Nonetheless, engrained dietary habits, lack of education about child care, cultural beliefs, and superstitions had to be overcome. To do so, the nurses had to "win the families' confidence."[48]

PRACTICING AT THE FULL EXTENT OF THEIR EDUCATION

In the camps the nurses worked at the full extent of their educational preparation. Present 9 a.m. to 5 p.m. every day, the nurses served as primary care providers, gate keepers, and physician extenders, working in collaboration with the local physicians who attended the clinics several mornings a week.[49] Nurses assessed each family member on admission and determined their needs. Protecting others in the camp from contagious diseases was as important as caring for the new arrivals, and if the nurse found that any member of the family had a communicable disease, she would assign him or her to "one of 10 to 12 isolation shelters" instead of the usual quarters.[50] Since physicians were in attendance only during specified hours a few times a week, the nurse had a "striking degree of responsibility," assessing patients, treating them according to standing order sets, triaging and referring them according to severity of illness.[51] More complicated cases were "referred to specialists, dentists, x-ray and clinical laboratories."[52] When a physician was in camp, the nurse returned to her more traditional role, assisting with simple medical treatments and minor surgeries, vaccinating patients, and giving medications.

More often than not, the camp nurse would diagnose and treat numerous common ailments on her own. Typically Mary Sears treated "impetigo, poison oak, scabies, dermatitis, and dietary deficiencies. She also dealt with epidemics of encephalitis and whooping cough, pink eye, trachoma," . . . as

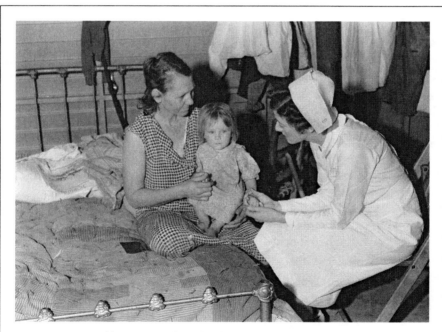

Nurse attending sick baby in migrant camp.

● ● ● ● ●

well as obstetric cases, tonsillitis, otitis media, and chronic diseases due to "lack of previous medical care."[53] One family case history illustrates the types of chronic diseases the nurses and physicians frequently encountered:

> The 41 year old mother had pellagra and dental caries along with uterine bleeding and anemia due to miscarriage; the father had "bad teeth" and "stomach pains"; The 15 year old daughter had "chronic tonsillitis," the 10 year old son had gastro-enteritis; and the 2 year old child had enlarged tonsils and an infected mosquito bite.[54]

Clearly, as one report noted, "neglect of chronic ailments" added up. In other instances, it seemed the more nurses saw and assessed patients, the more needs they identified. The case of a family from Castle, Oklahoma, who had come to California in 1937, is typical:

> . . . Mrs. C. applied for aid in June 1938 . . . asking for prenatal examination, confinement and post-natal care. Since the confinement, we have authorized treatment for an infected umbilicus in the infant and idiopathic diarrhea. . . . Our program is also treating the fifteen-year-old daughter for diabetes mellitus.[55]

Working with the migrants, the nurses merged their traditional starched image with the down-to-earth realities, expanding their time-honored role as handmaiden to the physician to include diagnosing and treating patients and providing care according to physician's standing orders.[56] As historian Michael Grey documented: "With the verbal approval of the camp doctor, [the nurses] could write prescriptions and dispense drugs from the clinic formulary."[57] They [also] staffed well-baby clinics, coordinated immunization programs, taught mothers about nutrition, and gave prenatal and postpartum care. On the other hand, they also continued in their customary work, making home visits to assess families' living conditions, giving direct bedside care, and teaching preventive health measures.

Sometimes, the nurse's role was more that of social worker than nurse; the lines blurred when it came to addressing the migrants' needs for shelter, clothes, blankets and food. Describing what she had done for the family living near the fence in the corner of the pea field, Mary Sears wrote:

> . . . There was nowhere to take them. I left a note for the parents—where to come for a tent and for surplus foods. . . . The family received a new tent, bedding, clothing and rations . . . and extensive medical care that included prescriptions from the grocery store for three high caloric diets . . . [58]

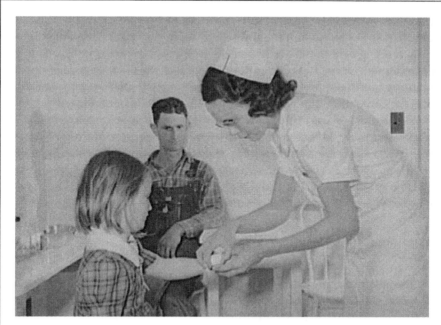

Nurse treating child in health clinic, Shafter migrant camp trailer.

● ● ● ● ●

The camp nurse's role also blurred with that of the nutritionist when it came to teaching the migrant mothers the basics of nutrition. Some young mothers didn't know much about food preparation outside of making biscuits and gravy, and needed to learn both the principles of a healthy diet and how to cook for their families.[59] Moreover, having access to government surplus foods did not necessarily solve their nutrition problems. In one case, even though the mother had powdered milk "given her off relief" from the government, she didn't use it. Her explanation to the nurse: "I don't guess I know how to mix it up." The nurse responded by demonstrating its preparation, and according to her report: "the two children devoured it voraciously."[60]

GAINING TRUST

Gaining the trust of the migrant community was essential if the nurse was to be an effective health care provider. The nurse also needed the community's help—there was simply too much for one person to do. To accomplish both objectives, in many of the camps the nurses organized committees of women who could report on those who were sick, ensure that the utility buildings (the location of showers, wash tubs, and toilets) were kept clean, and assist in providing nursing care for any sick member in the section of camp to which they were assigned. Often these committees served "as the nucleus to get women to attend the health conferences."[61] One migrant woman created a poster advertising the conference and attached it to the tree outside her tent.

Winning the trust of the migrant children was also important, and the nurses used both the art and science of nursing to do so. In one camp, the nurse used a "unique treatment" for children with pinkeye, one of the most contagious diseases she had to address. In this case, the nurse put "a drop of medicine in the child's eye and a piece of candy in the mouth." One healed; the other assured "further cooperation."[62]

FOLLOWING THE CROPS

Like the migrant families, the nurses followed the crops. It was, after all, important to be where the workers and their families were, and the nurses were constantly on the move. In the fall of 1939, for example, Mary Sears was sent to Marysville, 50 miles north of Sacramento, where an old camp was being replaced by a larger, much improved one near Yuba City. The new camp was not yet finished but the clinic was open for business. Sears also had responsibility for a small camp a few miles upriver and another in Winters, 60 miles away in the Sacramento Valley. She worked there only 1 day a week and referred patients to local doctors. As Sears recalled: "Life became busy sometimes even hectic; learning crops and problems in such a large new area, running a busy clinic and servicing two other camps."[63]

By 1939, there were 11 migratory labor camps scattered throughout California. By September 1941, there were 58 camps located across the United States, caring for about 160,000 people.[64] In the government camps, nurses had unprecedented responsibility and unprecedented autonomy. As one physician later recalled, "They were able to do a lot of what nurse practitioners do after a lot of training, but these nurses did it through experience."[65] Nursing supervisors agreed. In 1939, Olive Whitlock, director of the Division of Public Health Nursing for the Oregon State Board of Health, expressed her thoughts in a letter to the FSA regional office, writing that her chief concern was "over the amount of responsibility placed on the nurses."[66] Whitlock was probably correct in her assessment of the situation, but perhaps needless in her worry. Nurses used the full extent of their training, working at the limits of their scope of practice to meet the migrants' needs. They also recognized their professional boundaries and worked under physician supervision, albeit sometimes from a distance. Overall, the "government nurses" provided access to care for thousands of displaced and disenfranchised migratory laborers and their families.

CONCLUSION

The economic plight of predominantly White American migrant workers, the establishment of the AWHMA, and the acceptance of its programs by local medical societies all shaped the role public health nurses played during the Great Depression. In turn, the nurses played a central role in the health care workforce, entering the migrant camps as agents of the government, but working with a great deal of autonomy once there. The nurses' role was threefold: (1) to help the migrants keep healthy, (2) to keep migrants from spreading disease, and (3) to keep workers in the field. To do so, the nurses worked to the full extent of their education and preparation, at times blurring the professional boundaries among medicine, nursing, and social work. Through their actions and relationships with the migrants, the nurses raised the questions of whether or not access to health care was a right or a privilege, who was deserving of health care services, and who should make those decisions. Working within the social structure of the migrant community as well as cooperating with outside agencies such as the State Relief Association, the American Red Cross, and the Agriculture Workers Health and Medical Association, the nurses did what they could to meet the migrants' needs. Providing direct care as well as health teaching, the nurses who cared for the migrants questioned in action, if not in words, the "prevailing assumption that one's health was one's own responsibility."[67]

NOTES

1. Mary Sears, "The Nurse and the Migrant," *The Pacific Coast Journal of Nursing* 37, no. 3 (March 1941): 144–46 (quote, 145).

2. Michael R. Grey, "Dustbowls, Disease, and the New Deal: The Farm Security Administration Migrant Health Programs, 1935–1947," *The Journal of the History of Medicine and Allied Sciences, Inc.* 48 (1993): 3–39 (quote, 3).

3. Adam Cohen, *Nothing to Fear: FDR's Inner Circle and the Hundred Days that Created Modern America* (New York, NY: Penguin Books, 2009), 14.

4. Timothy Egan, *The Worst Hard Time: The Untold Story of Those Who Survived the Great American Depression* (New York, NY: Houghton Mifflin Harcourt, 2006).

5. Adam Cohen, *Nothing to Fear*, 16.

6. Russell Freedman, *Children of the Great Depression* (New York, NY: Clarion Books, 2005), 63.

7. Franklin D. Roosevelt, Second Inaugural Address, 1937.

8. Wanda D. Mann, "Migrant Nursing," *The Pacific Coast Journal of Nursing* 37, 11 (November, 1941): 658–60 (quote, 658).

9. Grey, "Dustbowls, Disease," 3–39 (quote, 10).

10. California State Relief Administration Report, Hollenberg Collection, Bancroft Library (hereafter cited as HC, BL) carton 2, pamphlet, one page.

11. California State Relief, Hollenberg Collection, one page.

12. FSA, *Migrant Farm Labor: The Problem and Some Efforts to Meet It,* pamphlet, HC, BL, no page.

13. Grey, "Dustbowls, Disease," 7.

14. Russell Freedman, *Children of the Great Depression*, 65.

15. FSA, *Migrant Farm Labor: The Problem and Some Efforts to Meet It,* pamphlet, 1937, HC, BL, no page.

16. FSA, *Migrant Farm Labor,* no page.

17. Ralph Williams, "Nursing Care for Migrant Families," *American Journal of Nursing* 41, no. 9 (1941): 1028–1032, (quote, 1030).

18. Sears, "The Nurse and the Migrant," 145.

19. Grey, "Dustbowls, Disease," 9.

20. FSA Programs: "The FSA's Low Cost Medical Program," 1937, p. 1, folder 2:1, carton 2, HC, BL.

21. Anita Faverman, Edna Rockstroh, Freda Whyte, and Laura Bolt, "Trailing Child and Maternal Health into California Migratory Agricultural Camps," *Report of the Second Year of the Migratory Demonstration, Nurses' Report* (July 1937–June 1938): 28–37 (quote, 36). HC, BL.

22. "Outline of Activities from March 4, 1938 to May 31, 1939," in Agriculture Worker Health and Medical Association, folder 2:1, carton 2, series 2 (programs) HC, BL, 1.

23. "Outline of Activities," in Agriculture Worker Health and Medical Association, HC, BL, 1.

24. Laura Bolt (nutritionist), "Nutritionist's Report," in Anita Faverman et al., "Trailing Child and Maternal Health," 1, 28–38.

25. FSA Case Report, (1938) HC, BL, carton 2, folder 2-11, one page.

26. "Report on Arvin and Shafter Camp Conditions," HC, BL.

27. Williams, "Nursing Care," (1941): 1031.

28. Williams, "Nursing Care," (1941): 1031.

29. Williams, "Nursing Care," (1941): 1031.

30. Omer Mills, "Health Problems among Migratory Workers" (U.S. Department of Agriculture, Region IX) (speech, annual convention of the California League of Municipalities, Santa Barbara, CA, September 8, 1938): 1–4 (quote, 4) HC, BL.

31. Sears, "The Nurse and the Migrant," 144–45.

32. Grey, "Dustbowls, Diseases," 11.

33. Faverman et al., "Trailing Child and Maternal Health," 28–37 (quote, 32).

34. Faverman et al., "Trailing Child and Maternal Health," 32.

35. Faverman et al., "Trailing Child and Maternal Health," 33

36. Faverman et al., "Trailing Child and Maternal Health," 30.

37. Faverman et al., "Trailing Child and Maternal Health," 31.

38. Faverman et al., "Trailing Child and Maternal Health," 29.

39. FSA, *Migrant Farm Labor: The Problem,* HC, BL, 15.

40. Charles Todd, "Trampling out the Vintage," *Common Sense.* (July 1939): 7–8 (quote, 7), accessed December 27, 2013, http://memory.loc.gov/egi-bin/ampage.

41. Faverman et al., "Trailing Child and Maternal Health," 34.

42. Faverman et al., "Trailing Child and Maternal Health," 35.

43. Eric Thomsen (Assistant Regional Director in Charge of California Migrant Labor Camps). "Migratory Labor–Asset or Liability" (speech, Bakersfield Rotary Club, July 29, 1938): 1–14 (quote, 5).

44. "A Medical Clinic on Wheels: The FSA Mobile Camps and Clinics for Migratory Workers," U.S. Department of Agriculture, FSA, Division of Information, Region IX, RG 389, box 2, folder 22 (May 1939): 1–3 (quote, 1).

45. Report on Camp at Arvin, California, no date, no author, carton 2, HC, BL.

46. Report on Camp, carton 2, HC, BL.

47. Mary Sears, "The Flat-Tired, Flat-Tired-People," "Voices from the Past," in Anne Loftis (ed.), *The Californians* (March–August 1989): 14–17, 58.

48. Williams, "Nursing Care," (1941): 1032.

49. Wanda Mann, "Migrant Nursing," 658.

50. Williams, "Nursing Care," 1030.

51. Grey, "Dustbowls, Diseases," 18.

52. Sears, "The Nurse and the Migrant," 145.

53. "Outline of Activities" in Agriculture Worker Health and Medical Association, HC, BL, 7.

54. FSA Case report, (no number), carton 2, folder 2, pp. 1–5 (quote, 1) HC, BL.

55. FSA Case report, 43, carton 2, folder 2, HC, BL.

56. Wanda D. Mann, "Migrant Nursing," 658.

57. Michael Grey, *New Deal Medicine: The Rural Health Programs of the Farm Security Administration* (Baltimore, MD: Johns Hopkins University Press, 1999), 94.

58. Sears, "The Flat-Tired, Flat-Tired-People," 14–17, 58, (quote, 15).

59. Omer Mills, "Health Problems among Migratory Workers" (U.S. Department of Agriculture, Region IX) (speech, annual convention of the California League of Municipalities, Santa Barbara, CA, September 8, 1938): 1–4. HC, BL.

60. Faverman et al., "Trailing Child and Maternal Health," 38.

61. Williams, "Nursing Care," (1941): 1032.

62. Williams, "Nursing Care," (1941): 1032.

63. Sears, "The Flat-Tired, Flat-Tired," 16.

64. Williams, "Nursing Care," (1941): 1029.

65. Grey, *New Deal Medicine*, 96.

66. Olive Whitlock, letter to Pearl McIver, Senior Public Health Nurse, 22 September 1941, NARA, Region X, Seattle, Washington.

67. Patricia D'Antonio (personal communication with author), January 18, 2014.

8

•••••

Nursing in West Texas:
Trains, Tumbleweeds, and Rattlesnakes

•••••

MELISSA McINTIRE SHERROD

I only did what I needed to do. It was frontier medicine and we just
made do with what we had and people depended on us. . . . It wasn't
like it is today . . . The state didn't make it better, so we had no choice.[1]

DURING AN INTERVIEW IN 2009, Judy Sherrod reflected on her experience
working with rural residents in the Trans-Pecos region of Texas during the oil
boom in the late 1940s. On the frontier she had had only her husband, herself,
and her training on which to rely. Judy was a bachelor's-prepared registered
nurse who had experience in administration and surgical nursing, and, as
she noted, she used "every bit of her knowledge, skill and experience" to handle life on the frontier. Working with her physician husband, Judy provided
access to care for thousands of Texans living in a remote region of west Texas,
an area booming with oil wells, bad water, tumbleweeds, and rattlesnakes.

EXPLORING THE PECOS

The Trans-Pecos, in far west Texas, is a 17,000 square mile region unlike any other
in the state. It is a place of extremes, a region distinguished by what it lacks—
water, timber, and people—and by its undefinable terrain. It's a region that cannot be classified as a plain, a plateau, as mountainous, or as desert because it is
all of these. The Pueblo Indians, who once lived along the banks of the upper
Pecos River, gave their name to the river.[2] The area lies west of the Pecos River
and is bound on the north by New Mexico and on the south by the Rio Grande.

In the early 19th century, the Trans-Pecos region was an effective barrier to the westward movement of Texas settlers. Settlers considered the region a barren and useless wasteland, a crossing to be endured until the land on the other side proved to be better. Water and timber were not easily obtained. Moreover, the local water was described as "a mixture of slimy saltiness, as if salt had been melted in soapy water; next a faint sweetness, followed by a distinct bitter, finally winding up with a distinct taste of lye."[3] The water was so bad that "coffee boiled in it" was described as "a villainous concoction."[4] Because of the scarcity of natural resources, the harshness of the land and few passable roads, the Trans-Pecos region would not be settled until much later.

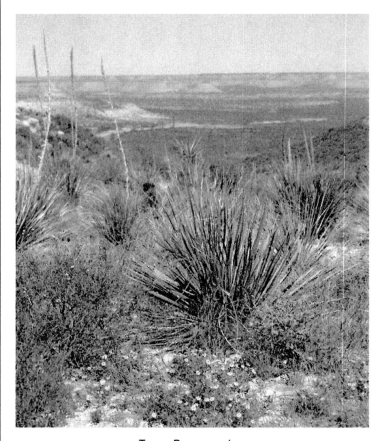

Trans-Pecos region.
Source: Photo courtesy of Melissa Sherrod.

● ● ● ● ●

RANCHING AND THE RAILROAD

Gradually, throughout the late-19th century, ranchers did arrive and settle the Trans-Pecos. By 1900 the area's population had increased to 2,360. County records noted 95 ranches and farms, encompassing 2,159,000 acres.[5] Cattle and sheep ranching dominated economic activity along with some oil prospecting. However, by 1910 the number of farms and ranches in the county had declined, and the population decreased to 2,071.[6] In 1913, construction of a railroad across Pecos County by the Kansas City, Mexico and Orient Railway Company caused a boom in land speculation and community growth. New irrigation projects along the Pecos River in the northern part of the county also began to attract land buyers. By 1920 there were 207 farms and ranches in the area. Eight thousand acres were planted in cotton with another 534 acres planted in sorghum. However, during the Great Depression, growth declined when the farmers in Pecos County lost their land and livelihoods to drought and foreclosure. By 1940 only 326 farms and ranches remained in the county.

TEXAS TEA

Oil prospecting began in Pecos County in 1900. "Texas tea" had previously been discovered in other parts of Texas, but it was thought that oil could not be found west of the Pecos River, an area described as one that "even buffalo know better than to cross."[7] The discovery of oil in Pecos County in 1926 dramatically changed the region economically and socially.

In the early 1920s, Mr. Ira Yates, an entrepreneur and rancher, was struggling to make his ranch profitable. He approached the Mid-Kansas Oil Company and the Transcontinental Oil Company and convinced them to drill on his ranch despite its location in the Trans-Pecos region. On October 26, 1926, the Mid-Kansas Oil and Gas Company and the Transcontinental Oil Company drilled the first well on Yates's land. Yates shared the lease with the oil companies and together they drilled four wells. On the fourth try they drilled an exploratory oil well, known as Yates 1, to a depth of 1,005 feet and hit a gusher. Each successive well yielded a similar result and Ira Yates became an instant millionaire. Production of Yates's oil field peaked in 1929 with a total output of 41 million barrels of oil. That year, an oil well named Yates 3 produced 8,325 barrels per hour and 200,000 barrels a day.[8]

When the oil field was discovered, workers arrived from around the country, creating an instant boomtown. The town, named Redbarn, was populated with workers who lived in tents and hastily built shanties around the perimeter of the oil field. At its peak, the town's population totaled

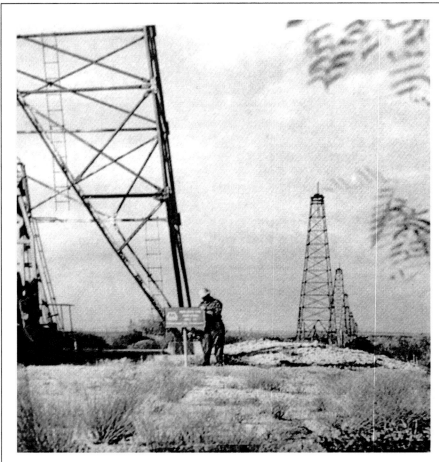

Yates Field #1.

● ● ● ● ●

75 residents. In 1926, Ira Yates donated 152 acres of his ranch 3 miles north of Redbarn to create the town of Iraan. Oil companies rushed to move workers and their families to the new town. The Ohio Oil Company, majority owner of the drilling rights to Yates's field, built company houses and drilled wells for water. A year later, in 1927, they constructed a school and hired teachers. By 1928 the town opened its own post office. Within 4 years of being established, Iraan had 60 businesses and an estimated population of 1,600 residents.[9]

Providing health care to Iraan's residents was a challenge. Only one doctor, Marvin Greer Rape, MD, and a few nurses were available for the entire area. The closest hospital was in Fort Stockton, 65 miles away. It was a challenging distance due to poor road conditions and the lack of transportation, especially when acutely ill or injured citizens needed medical services. Isolation and the dangerous work associated with ranches and oil rigs left the residents of Pecos County particularly vulnerable. In addition, the few resources that existed were strained by the lack of state funding and services.[10]

THE EARLY WEST TEXAS OIL INDUSTRY

In the early days of oil exploration, environmental controls were at best lax, at worst nonexistent. Poorly constructed wells leaked crude oil. The unsealed portions of the well casing—metal pipe used to shore up the structure and sides of the well hole—oozed oil that seeped up through the soil, contaminating the Pecos River. Indeed, the leakage was so extreme that it was possible to skim off thousands of barrels of oil per day from the river. The lack of transportation, storage facilities, and any formal infrastructure made transporting the crude oil an impossible task. As a result of the tremendous output of the field and insufficient containment, oil leaked into the ground and into nearby canyons. By mid-1933, over 3.25 million barrels of seepage oil had been gathered. Meanwhile, oil production in Yates's oil fields climbed to over 13 million barrels in 1945 and to more than 18 million by 1948.[11]

ROUGHNECKS AND RATTLESNAKES

"When I think of the oil patch, I don't think of music."[12] These were the words of Elmer Kelton, an award-winning Western novelist from Crane, Texas, during the 1920s oil boom days. While country music was popular in other industrial areas in the South and the West, songs about the Texas oil fields did not find wide acceptance. According to music historian Bill Malone, the reason for this lack of interest was the absence of a sense of community. Crews seldom stayed together for extended periods of time. Compared to the romantic images of the open range with cowboys on horseback serenading the herd or singing by the campfire, the images of life in the oil field were ugly. Working an oilrig was dirty, difficult, and dangerous. The constant noise of the drilling operation did little "to encourage conversation, [much] less singing," noted folklorist Mody Boatright.[13] There was no time for daydreaming in the oil fields; lack of complete concentration could result in serious injury or death.

Several oil companies had interests in Yates's field, chief among them the Ohio Oil Company and the Marathon Oil Company. Workers from across the United States, also interested in Yates's oil field, came from Pennsylvania, Ohio, Illinois, California, and Louisiana, as well as Texas. Due to the transient nature of the job, thousands of workers known as "roustabouts" drifted through the region during the boom. While some workers brought their wives and children, others came alone and lived in company bunkhouses or temporary housing.

Over time, however, increasing numbers of women came to west Texas. They frequently lived in oil camps or in "shotgun" houses with dirt floors. Sand storms proved a constant threat, as did the harsh environment. Raising small children was particularly difficult. One young mother noted that her baby learned to walk in his crib because she didn't want him to walk on the dirt floor where rattlesnakes, tarantulas, and scorpions[14] were a threat.

Despite these difficulties, the tiny community of Iraan continued to experience major growth. The need for a more stable community prompted the building of schools, churches, and community buildings and was made possible by support from area oil company executives, businessmen, ministers, and their church groups.[15] By 1940, Yates's field, while diminished in oil production from the early days, was still a major employer in the region and continued to contribute to regional and economic growth.[16]

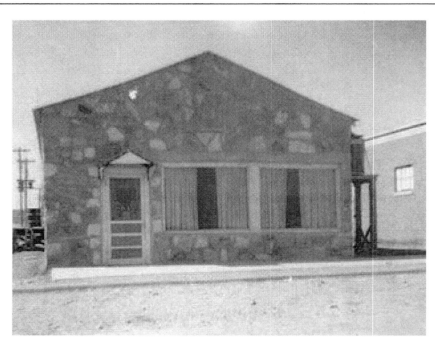

First Iraan office.
Source: Photo courtesy of Melissa Sherrod.

• • • • •

"LIKE A WAR ZONE"

As a result of lax industrial safety standards, oil field accidents comprised a major cause of death in the region. The lack of accessible medical services also contributed to the mortality figures. One incident stands out. In March 1949, the *Iraan News* reported the death of a local driller when he was struck by falling machinery on the Gulf-Yates lease west of Iraan. According to the report, members of the crew were attempting to set up a rig at the time the accident occurred. The man "was pinned under the fallen rig. As the rest of the crew attempted to gain his release, a container of acid burst and spilled on the injured man while he was pinned underneath the machinery."[17] Even though he was given first aid treatment at the scene, the patient died en route to a San Angelo Hospital, some 90 miles away.[18]

Besides the employees of the oil fields, those who lived and worked on ranches miles from town in Pecos County were also at risk for accidents and had to deal with the lack of accessible medical services. When accidents occurred on these remote ranches, transportation was particularly problematic; poorly maintained ranch roads made access to emergency medical care even more difficult when minutes could differentiate life from death. In one accident, a 10-year-old girl suffered serious burns to her lower body while standing too near a campfire on her family's ranch, which was 20 miles from the closest town. The *Iraan News* reported that she received second- and third-degree burns when a "boy who was working on the ranch was attending to a fire where they were barbecuing in the backyard. He picked up a can with gasoline and poured it on the fire, causing the can to ignite. In his excitement he threw the can and hit the child. She was severely burned on her legs and thighs. She was admitted to the Crane Memorial Hospital and then was transferred to San Angelo the next day."[19]

Automobile accidents increasingly became a major cause of injury and death as the county's population grew and road improvement lagged behind. All of the two-lane roads in the county covered long open stretches of land, making it common to drive as fast as the cars allowed. While most of the terrain was flat, some areas were hilly with steep embankments. Slow-moving oil trucks along these stretches were always a concern, especially in the hills where visibility was limited. A fatal accident along one of these roads was particularly devastating to the residents of the small town. A story in the *Iraan News* told of the untimely death of a local son killed in an automobile accident "two miles north of Sheffield on the Old Spanish Trail." An approaching car on the curve was determined to be the immediate cause of the wreck; the car spun out of control, "overturning several times as it went over the embankment of the curve."[20]

As a result of an increasing number of accidents, local business leaders decided that the community needed to attract a new doctor. The lone physician in the community was elderly and many were concerned that he was unable to provide the necessary care for the increasing number of trauma victims in the community. Few physicians wanted to come to this part of Texas. If the community could even attract a physician, the residents rightfully assumed that as soon as the doctor's wife saw the hard scrabble community and the lack of an upscale social life, he would immediately reject any offer. Frank G. Bascom, the superintendent of the Ohio Oil Company, however, knew a young doctor who would soon be looking for a place to start a practice. Bascom's wife had a nephew who was finishing a surgical residency in St. Louis and Bascom considered him to be just what the town needed. Plus, the Ohio Oil Company was willing to make the offer an attractive one.

AN OFFER ACCEPTED

With the community leaders' support, Bascom wrote to his nephew, inviting the young doctor and his wife to visit the town and meet the local residents and community leaders. The couple was offered, free of charge, an updated office furnished with all the supplies they needed to begin practicing medicine. Bascom would provide the family transportation to Iraan; in addition, all of their belongings would be shipped to town at no cost to them.[21] It was an offer that Alan and Judy Sherrod could not refuse. As the *Iraan News* reported in August 1949:

> Dr. Allen Sherrod and family are expected this week. The Sherrods will make their home in Iraan, where Dr. Sherrod will engage in medical practice. Having visited Iraan sometime last winter, the Sherrods are quite enthused over the town and climate and are returning to make Iraan their home. Dr. Sherrod will begin practice as soon as his office is completed. He is a medical surgeon and general practitioner and comes to Iraan very highly recommended by his former associates.[22]

The call from Frank Bascom to Sherrod came just in time. As a senior resident surgeon at the Missouri Pacific Hospital, Alan Sherrod's duties would end on June 30, 1949. He had a wife and three children to support, and no idea how he was going manage. In addition, he was recovering from tuberculosis and had been advised to relocate to an arid region.[23] In fact, in 1944 Dr. Sherrod had had experimental surgery in which his affected lung and three ribs had been removed. He had recovered with Judy's help and began his surgical residency with the Missouri Pacific Hospital in May 1946. The couple's experience with fighting tuberculosis proved to be the foundation for the rest of their professional lives: they both recognized the importance of health promotion and health education within the community as the first line of defense against communicable diseases.[24]

A NEW LIFE IN WEST TEXAS

The Sherrods left St. Louis in August of 1949 and traveled to Midland, Texas, by train with three young children, all of their belongings, and virtually no savings. Once they arrived in Midland, they were met by Alan's uncle, Frank Bascom, and driven to Iraan some 90 miles south. In her book, *Independence Creek: The Story of a Texas Ranch*, Charlena Chandler writes about the community during the time:

> A spirit of relaxation and camaraderie usually prevailed among the people. In almost all respects, they were equal: their Anglo-American background was the same, as were also their social standards and ways of life. In a sense, they formed one large family, open and friendly in their relations, enjoying the freedoms of a frontier society, stimulated by the daily news of gushers coming in and wealth being produced in abundance.[25]

The oil boom was almost finished by the end of the 1940s, but a community spirit remained. There was little social hierarchy as far as what the men did for a living. Practically everyone depended on Yates's field for an income. Most wage earners, many of whom were transients who followed the rigs, worked for one of the many drilling companies or for small businesses supported by the oil field.[26] What was not said, however, was that the town was segregated racially. It was the South in the first half of the 20th century, and a Jim Crow society prevailed.

Other than a few teachers at the Iraan public school, few married women had jobs outside of the home. Most were not expected to bring in a second income and it was considered unusual if they did. Most of the wives were involved in local church and school activities, and organized community pageants and programs. When Alan and Judy Sherrod arrived in Iraan in the summer of 1949, Judy immediately went to work setting up the office, keeping the books, ordering supplies, and assisting with patients as needed. While this was considered odd, most of the people in town knew that Judy was a nurse and highly trained as a surgical assistant.

The first day Dr. Sherrod's office opened in September of 1949, 95 people lined up outside his door for care. Judy remembers looking out the door wondering what they were going to do for all of them. Each day was the same. She tried to get the townspeople to make appointments, but they were so unaccustomed to calling ahead that she finally decided to take them on a first-come, first-served basis. While the office was usually filled with patients, Alan often found himself treating trauma victims in the community as well. His medical training during his residency in St. Louis made him well prepared to care for these victims. Having been specifically trained to operate at the war front, Alan easily handled the common injuries: crush injuries, blast injuries, and amputations. Alan often commented that he and Judy often treated injuries that looked like war wounds.[27]

To complicate matters, much of the care they delivered occurred on ranches, on drilling sites, on roadways, or in fields with no easy access. While Alan traveled to a drilling site or from ranch to ranch seeing families and their ranch hands, Judy remained in town to see patients in the office. Eventually the Sherrods hired another registered nurse to manage the clinic workflow, but much of the time Judy stayed in the office, suturing lacerations, giving injections, writing prescriptions, and bandaging open wounds. When asked if she was concerned at the time that someone would think she was practicing medicine, Judy responded, "No, of course not. I knew what Alan would have done and what he would want me to do. I was trained in the OR and he showed me how to suture, set broken bones, and debride wounds. I was just doing what he would want me to do." But when asked how she gave prescriptions to patients who needed antibiotics or other medications, she commented, "You know, I wasn't prescribing medicine for people. I had a prescription pad that was stamped with his name on it, and I knew what to give the patients. I was very aware of what they needed and what Alan would want me to give them. Besides, I was knowledgeable about pharmacology as a nurse. I was just doing what I had to do under the circumstances. There was no one else to do it."[28]

Patients frequently called Dr. Sherrod at his house, regardless of the time of day or night. In one account, according to Charlena Chandler, an accident occurred at her father's ranch one evening. A group of high school students from Crane went to the ranch for an outing. "Several of the young men had gone hiking and as darkness fell, one of them separated from his friends to take a shortcut. No one actually saw his fall, but he fell from one of the lower bluffs on the (Pecos) river. He was mortally injured. My dad knew he could not be moved so we sent for family to stay at the scene while he drove to Iraan to get medical help. When Dad returned, after carrying Dr. Sherrod across the river piggyback, he was pronounced dead."[29]

ADDRESSING COMMUNITY NEEDS

In the late 1940s, Iraan was in dire need of health promotion and prevention programs. The Sherrods addressed the issue along with their other work. When Judy wasn't in the office, she was busy working in the community on public health projects. She assisted her husband, who had been appointed as the county health officer, or worked on her own initiatives. The pair quickly organized a series of community events aimed at preventing disease. There was little in the way of state funding for public health programs and most of the care at the time was achieved with community involvement. Officials in Austin reported the incidence of disease and would travel around the state to inform community leaders of any specific threat, but they depended on those in the community to raise awareness, organize fund raising drives, and get people out for screening events.

Health officials in Iraan, like those in other parts of the country, were concerned about the spread of tuberculosis, polio, chickenpox, measles, mumps, and whooping cough. The State Health Department suggested that civic groups in the community become involved to organize and fund public health programs. The Department pointed out that the "full support of each community will be necessary to make a difference."[30] In late 1949, the Health Department made plans for a mass chest x-ray survey of Pecos County to screen for tuberculosis. Over a 3-day period, 795 people over the age of 15 were x-rayed.[31]

The Sherrods made a major contribution to the state's public health efforts. Judy became involved in screening efforts in the office. She also helped as a community leader, working to immunize and educate office patients. Alan made house calls to all of the ranches in the county, immunizing many of the ranchers, workers, and their families. Nonetheless, Judy was determined that more needed to be done if they were to reach everyone.[32]

In 1953, Iraan held its first public immunization drive in the Civic Center. Judy had conceived of the idea based on her work in the community and the stories Alan had told about the lives of the itinerant workers on area ranches. She talked with pharmaceutical representatives who came by the office and wrote letters to their corporate offices asking for free vaccines. Turning to the Women's Auxiliary of the Big Bend Medical Society, an organization of which she was a member, Judy convinced the organization's leaders to make the immunization clinic a major fund raising activity. The town of Iraan gave the use of the community center. Later, other clinics were held in nearby Sheffield, a community of about 350 low-income Mexican workers and their families.[33]

Judy's goal was to immunize all of the children in the region, regardless of race, age, or family income. The cost was minimal for those who could pay, and free for those who could not. In one room of the center, Judy recorded health information and logged it into registries to be kept in the community. She administered immunizations and taught classes to mothers with small children and infants. The classes, taught in both English and Spanish, were intended to improve hygiene in the home; provide advice on infant feeding, growth, and development; and educate the mothers on the importance of immunizing everyone in the family. Dr. Sherrod gave general examinations, weighed and measured the infants and children, and checked them for symptoms of disease. The monthly clinics were a success: families came for routine medical screening and to immunize their children at no cost. The Sherrods' kindness to the Spanish-speaking community did not go unnoticed, nor did it go unnoticed by the state when, several years later, a representative from the Texas State Health Department came to Pecos County to help immunize the children in the region.[34] Town leaders told the representative that the state's help wasn't needed: The local doctor and nurse had immunized all the children.[35]

POLIO IN THE TRANS-PECOS

In the late 1940s, the United States was in the grip of a polio epidemic that could not be controlled. Reports of polio cases in Texas were soon widespread. In 1948 the *Iraan News* reported that there were 1,725 cases of polio in the state. By 1949 the number increased to 2,323.[36] The March of Dimes provided emergency funding to help defray the costs of immunizations and care for polio victims. Meanwhile, in Iraan Judy Sherrod was part of an effort to encourage people to donate money and to hold benefit basketball and volleyball games to aid in the cause.

It soon became clear that controlling the polio epidemic and caring for the victims would take the effort of several organizations, not just the efforts of the state health department and the Sherrods. The local Lions Club did its part and arranged a polio "cleanup" campaign to keep Iraan free of the disease. An article in the local newspaper instructed residents "to clean your premises of tin cans, bottles, old tires, weeds and other trash. Check your out-door toilets. Our state law says they should be fly proof. Eliminate flies, rats and mosquitoes, as well as fire hazards. Soon after Iraan is cleaned up, it will be sprayed with D.D.T."[37]

As the fight against polio continued, more national, state, and regional organizations became involved in preventing and managing this dreaded disease. By the early 1950s, the citizens of Iraan were asked to donate blood to the Red Cross to create a supply of gamma globulin to fight the polio epidemic. Judy was the chairman of the Iraan blood drive. The Women's

Auxiliary to the Big Bend Medical Society sponsored the drive, which included the Texas counties of Pecos, Jeff Davis, Brewster, and Presidio, an area that covered over 17,000 square miles. Judy announced that the oil companies, as well as civic and church groups, had helped to obtain transportation to the blood mobile for many of the area's citizens.

In 1951 the Sherrods' son Peter contracted polio while on vacation in St. Louis. The *Iraan News* reported that initially he was almost completely paralyzed and an iron lung was available in his hospital room in case it was needed. With rehabilitation and good nursing care provided in the hospital and at home, Peter gradually recovered. After personally experiencing the dreaded disease, Judy committed her time to the community, organizing fund raising drives and working to keep the community informed of the most current information available on polio.[38]

CHALLENGING EMERGENCY TRANSPORTS

The vast expanses of Texas, the shortage of physicians, the lack of ambulance facilities, and rough roads proved to be continuous challenges for the Sherrods as they tried to meet patient needs in the isolated Trans-Pecos area. Almost every day Dr. Alan Sherrod drove 120 miles round trip to Fort Stockton and back in order to see his patients or to perform surgeries in the local hospital. One day while Alan was away from his office, working in Fort Stockton, one of the oil rig workers fell and was seriously injured. Concerned that their fellow worker had possibly broken his back, several workers took the injured man to the Sherrods' office in Iraan. Although Alan was not there, Judy quickly assessed the victim and realized immediately that he would have to be immobilized for transport to the hospital in Fort Stockton. Thinking fast, she grabbed the only apparatus for immobilization that she had—her ironing board. Judy directed the men to place the patient on the board and carefully place it on the back seat of her car. She then drove to Fort Stockton where Alan and other physicians attended to the patient's injuries. It was simple: Judy worked with what she had to do whatever needed to be done.

This was not the only time Judy transported critically ill patients to Fort Stockton. Her son remembers many similar incidents in which he was a passenger. He recalls, "Those big ol' cars then could go really fast. I remember she'd be going about 100 miles an hour down those two lane roads, and the suspension in those cars was really soft so it felt like you were in the ocean kind of floating over the bumps. It made me go to sleep but it was probably good for all those people she transported."[39]

CONCLUSION

By the late 1940s, many of the farms and ranches in the Trans-Pecos had been sold due to the effects of the Great Depression and a series of droughts. The region was in the midst of a decades-long oil boom that brought workers from all around the country. The work was dangerous and industrial safety standards were virtually nonexistent. Oil crews seldom stayed on the job long and drifted from one oil rig to another. Lacking a sense of community, roughnecks were known as independent, free-spirited transients who lived for a short time in company-owned camps, but did not put down roots. Eventually the oil companies built and funded communities in an effort to attract company managers and their families to the area. The gravity of some of the accidents associated with oil drilling and ranching was compounded by the isolation of the region and the lack of access to care, geographically, economically, and culturally.

Life in the oil town of Iraan during the late 1940s was intricately ordered. The intermixing of social culture and traditions was met outwardly with community acceptance. Health care needs and health drives were regarded as a community effort, to be supported by all regardless of race, occupation, or position in the social hierarchy. The Sherrods, the only nurse and doctor in 800 square miles, acted according to their faith, their belief in social justice, and the necessity of using sound scientific principles to guide their professional care. Because of the extreme need for health care providers, Judy Sherrod worked to the fullest extent of her education and experience, providing health care to patients in town, residents on ranches in the county, and to all of the citizens in the Trans-Pecos region. In an effort to reduce infant mortality and improve the lives of area families when services were not provided by state or local authorities, she independently acted to bring immunizations and education to hundreds of impoverished Mexican and White women and children from the ranches and oil camps in the area, as well as the citizens in town. Responding to immediate health care needs, she met each challenge with strength and determination, using logic and information to devise a plan and execute it with care. In so doing, she brought much-needed information, expertise, and skill to a diverse population that would have been denied care in an isolated corner of west Texas.

NOTES

1. Judy Sherrod, interview in 2009 by Melissa Sherrod.

2. J.P. Burnett, Trans-Pecos Texas: A Study of Exploration (Rockwall, TX, Texas A & I University, 1970, 4). The name Pecos belongs to the Qq'ueres language, the language of the Pueblo, and is pronounced Pae-qp. The first mention of the name Pecos

is found in documents dated 1598 after a general meeting of Juan de Onate, a Spanish explorer, with the Pueblo Indians in the Estufa or Pueblo of Santa Domingo.

3. Colonel Nathanial Alston Taylor, *The Coming Empire of Two Thousand Miles in Texas on Horseback* (Houston, TX: N. T. Carlisle, 1936), 299–300.

4. Taylor, *Coming Empire of Two Thousand Miles*, 299–300.

5. Glenn Justice and John Leffler, "Pecos County," Handbook of Texas Online, accessed November 1, 2013, http://www.tshaonline.org/handbook/online/articles/hcp05, Published by the Texas State Historical Association.

6. Justice and Leffler, "Pecos County," November 1, 2013.

7. J. J. Bowden, Uncertain Riches: The Discovery and Exploitation of the Yates Oil Field (Austin, TX: Eakin Press, 1991), 49.

8. D. D. Hinton and R. M. Olien, Oil in Texas: The Gusher Age 1895–1945, (Austin, TX: University of Texas Press, 2002).

9. Pecos County Historical Commission, Pecos County History, vol. 2 (Canyon, TX: Staked Plains, 1984).

10. Pecos County Historical Commission, Pecos County History, 1984.

11. Julia Cauble Smith, "Yates Oilfied," Handbook of Texas Online, accessed November 12, 2013, http://www.tshaonline.org/handbook/online/articles/doy01, Published by the Texas State Historical Association.

12. Joe Specht, "I'm a Tool Pusher from Snyder: Slim Willet's Oil Patch Songs," Southwestern Historical Quarterly 113, no. 3:293–309.

13. Specht, "I'm a Tool Pusher from Snyder," 294.

14. Pauline Boles, interview in 1985.

15. Glenn Justice, "Iraan, TX," Handbook of Texas Online, accessed November 12, 2013. http://www.tshaonline.org/handbook/online/articles/hji02, Published by the Texas State Historical Association.

16. The population of Iraan was listed in the U.S. Census in 1940 as 1,907, with another 324 in nearby Sheffield and Bakersfield.

17. The *Iraan News*, "Driller Fatally Injured in Industrial Accident Wednesday," March 25, 1949.

18. The *Iraan News*, March 25, 1949.

19. The *Iraan News*, "Local Rancher's Daughter Suffers Burns in Accident at Ranch Tuesday Night," July 10, 1951.

20. The *Iraan News*, "Iraanite Killed in Car Accident Near Sheffield Last Friday Night," March 9, 1951.

21. Alan Sherrod, interview in 1996 by Melissa Sherrod.

22. The *Iraan News*, "Dr. Allen Sherrod to Open Office Here Soon," August 12, 1949.

23. Alan Sherrod, interview in 1996 by Melissa Sherrod.

24. Judy Sherrod, interview in 1996 by Melissa Sherrod.

25. Charlena Chandler, *Independence Creek: The Story of a Texas Ranch* (Lubbock, TX: Texas Tech University Press, 2004), 107.

26. Chandler, *Independence Creek*, 109–110.

27. Judy and Alan Sherrod, interview in 2003 by Melissa Sherrod.

28. Judy Sherrod, interview in 2009 by Melissa Sherrod.

29. Chandler, *Independence Creek*, 127.

30. The *Iraan News*, "Mass Chest X-Ray Survey To Be Taken In Pecos County," March 1, 1949.

31. The *Iraan News*, "Mass X-Ray Hailed as 'Successful' Here," March 12, 1949.

32. Judy Sherrod, interview in 1996 by Melissa Sherrod.

33. The *Iraan News*, "County Immunization Drive Underway this Week," March 26, 1952.

34. Family members noted that when they went to church or were met in public, many would bow or try to kiss their hands, or touch their arms as a gesture of thanks. For some, their presence in the community was seen as an omen of good fortune.

35. Judy Sherrod, interview in 1996 by Melissa Sherrod.

36. The *Iraan News*, "March of Dimes Drive Continues In Iraan," January 27, 1950.

37. The *Iraan News*, "Polio Clean Up Campaign," June 24, 1949.

38. Peter was fortunate and recovered; his recovery was a credit to the exemplary nursing care and rehabilitation he received both while in the hospital and at home. The *Iraan News*, "Red Cross Bloodmobile In Ft. Stockton August 5," July 17, 1953.

39. Michael Sherrod, interview in November 2013 by Melissa Sherrod.

9

•••••

Nursing the Navajo:
Dust Storms and Gully Washouts

•••••

ARLENE W. KEELING

... When a rumor of a typhoid outbreak reached the hospital, I was asked to make as frequent visits as possible to the neighborhood to check on suspected cases. This I have done three times a week and in addition have been holding a clinic at the Trading Post, 90 miles in another direction, once a week. . . . The sun blazes and no tree offers shade, the dust flies in smothering clouds, and yet we dread the coming of the seasonal rains which either cause us to stick in the mud or wait for hours on the bank of a wash while the water goes down . . .[1]

WRITING ON AUGUST 1, 1932, Elizabeth Forster, a field nurse working for the Bureau of Indian Affairs (BIA), described the difficulties she experienced reaching her patients. Forster was stationed in a remote trading post in Red Rock, Arizona, on the Navajo reservation. Bounded by the Grand Canyon on the west and extending east into New Mexico, the reservation was mostly desert, sparsely dotted with buttes and rocks, pinon trees, and grasses.[2] Scattered over great distances throughout the reservation, the sheep-herding Navajo lived in one-room homes, called hogans, made of logs and mud.

For the field nurses, just reaching the Navajo people was difficult. Sometimes traveling alone and sometimes accompanied by Navajo drivers who also served as interpreters, the nurses crossed the barren landscape to make home visits, driving from 800 to 2,500 miles a month.[3] Travel in the summer monsoon season was especially difficult as torrential downpours often caused gully wash-outs. Sandstorms, high winds, and searing heat further complicated

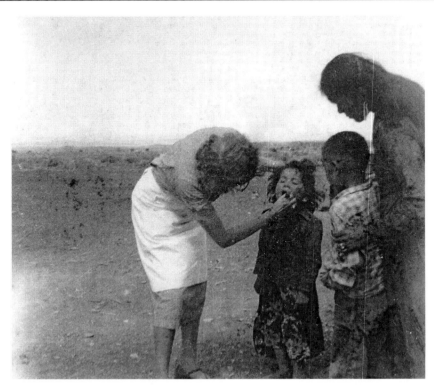

Ida Bahl examines Navajo girl, woman, and boy, 1955.

● ● ● ● ●

travel. In winter, blinding blizzards could close roads indefinitely.[4] The extreme weather, combined with great distances, poor roads, the lack of bridges, and the lack of any protection in the nurses' open-top Model T Fords, all created significant barriers to access to patients and families.[5] The challenges of crossing the borderlands of the Navajo culture and of incorporating their health beliefs and practices into the nurses' care were even more difficult.

In March 1936, field nurse Gladys Solverson reported her difficulties to the Bureau of Indian Affairs, writing:

This month we have had considerable illness on the reservation. 404 patients were visited and advised in their homes and 74 cases were seen at Trading Posts or Day Schools. We traveled 2025 miles and 110 hours over good and bad roads or more often, no road at all to reach these patients.[6]

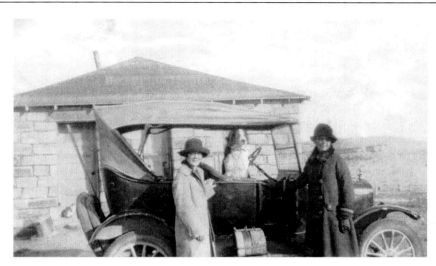

Elizabeth Foster with Model T Ford, 1925.

● ● ● ● ●

In addition to making home visits, the nurses conducted "nursing conferences" to instruct the Navajo women about infant and child care, sanitation,
nutrition, and the importance of prenatal care. The conferences were also for
the purpose of giving immunizations, making baby clothes, and conducting
well baby checkups. In May 1931, field nurse Dorothy Williams documented
some of the activities in a report of her work at Teec Nos Pas:

> Five clinics held this week, three general and two baby clinics. Mothers
> bathed their babies and were given material to cut out and make gowns
> for baby. Preschool children were weighed, inspected and mothers ad-
> vised [about] diets for underweights [sic] . . .

Reaching the isolated rural areas on the Navajo reservation to conduct the
clinics was not easy. When the roads were impassable or the nurses had car
trouble, scheduled clinics were often canceled.[7]

THE FEDERAL INITIATIVE

The nurses' work in the Four Corners Region (where Colorado, New Mexico,
Arizona, and Utah meet) was an experimental public health program sponsored by the New Mexico Association of Indian Affairs as part of a federal

government initiative to provide health care to American Indians on reservations throughout the United States. The initiative began in 1849 with the transfer of the BIA from the War Department to the Department of the Interior. However, from its inception, there were never enough doctors to meet the Indians' needs. Adding to that problem, there were no nurses. In fact, the BIA did not employ nurses until the 1890s, when they hired a few to work in the Indian boarding schools.[8]

By 1900, the BIA had built several hospitals and had increased the number of boarding schools on the reservations, but it was not until 1921 that Congress passed the Snyder Act, authorizing significant federal funds for health services to Native American tribes. Instead of using the funds to set up field clinics, the BIA built more hospitals. The problem was that the Navajo did not use hospitals. They believed death lay within the hospital walls and therefore the buildings were filled with evil spirits, *"Ch'iindis."*

In an attempt to better meet the Indians' needs, in 1922 the Office of Indian Affairs commissioned the American Red Cross to conduct a survey of the health needs on the reservations. Two years later, the Red Cross recommended "the immediate establishment of an organized public health nursing service as part of the Indian health program."[9] A pilot program, employing three trained Red Cross nurses as visiting nurses on the Navajo reservation, followed. The experiment was a success, but because of inadequate funding, it would take years to get the nursing service up and running.

THE *MERIAM REPORT* AND THE FIELD NURSES

In the mid-1920s, U.S. Secretary of the Interior Hubert Work commissioned Lewis Meriam, a medical specialist employed by the Department of the Interior, to conduct a survey of the health services provided to the American Indians. The results, published in 1928 in the *Meriam Report*, were graphic in detail, describing extreme poverty, poor health and nutrition, and a lack of sanitation among the Indians. In addition, the report documented inadequate salaries for physicians and nurses, inadequate medical facilities, and minimal efforts toward preventive medicine. It also confirmed the fact that the two "great health problems" continued to be tuberculosis and trachoma. According to the report, the Indian death rate from tuberculosis in Arizona was "15.1, more than seventeen times as high as the general rate for the country as a whole."[10]

COLLABORATION VERSUS AUTONOMOUS PRACTICE

Ideally, a physician–nurse pair worked together to provide care, often setting up clinics in areas where the Navajo were already meeting in order to give immunizations and provide health teaching. As field nurse Dorothy Williams noted:

> March 16–21, 1936: Four clinics held this week; large number of Navajo in for medicine and treatment. Dr. Elliott and myself [sic] attended the farmers meeting at Teec Nos Pas and he explained to the Navajo the reason for the children being vaccinated and having inoculation etc. and answered all the questions . . .[11]

Having a physician present at the clinics or in the home was the ideal rather than the reality. The chronic physician shortage, the vast distances, and the extreme weather conditions often resulted in the nurses working alone or accompanied only by their Navajo drivers. Field nurse Mary Eppich lamented the fact in one of her monthly reports, writing: "Have had several sick patients at the hogans and have wanted Dr. Stephenson to see them, but he has not made any clinics this month . . ."[12] When their Indian drivers were also unavailable, the nurses made home visits by themselves.[13]

Practicing under these conditions, the BIA nurses did whatever they had to do to care for the Navajo people. In April 1933, Elizabeth Forster saw 397 patients in her dispensary and made 65 hogan visits.[14] In May 1935, Nena Seymour made home visits to "76 different Hogans," treating "sore throats, ear infections, cuts, impetigo and other commonly occurring diseases."[15] Among the most widespread were trachoma, tuberculosis, and impetigo.

TRACHOMA

One of the most troublesome diseases that plagued the Navajo was trachoma, a highly contagious disease that ran rampant on the reservation. Aggravated by the hot desert climate as well as dust and wind, trachoma caused granular bumps on the inside of a patient's eyelids. When these scratched the cornea, the patient experienced excruciating pain. Left untreated, the disease eventually resulted in blindness.

So, in addition to holding the well-baby conferences and immunization clinics, the field nurses held specialty clinics to address the problem of trachoma, traveling to isolated areas of the reservation to do so. In one instance, field nurse Nena Seymour opened a "Community Medical Center" in the mountains to reach the Navajo who migrated there for the summer. Reporting on her work, Seymour noted:

> My Mexican Springs dispensary is at last painted and I set up clinics. Routine trachoma treatments have been started. I have set aside 7:30–9:00 am for trachoma treatments . . . each day.[16]

Realizing that the White man's medicine not only relieved their pain and itching, but also helped them preserve their eyesight, the ever-practical Navajo bypassed their traditional cures for the disease and willingly attended the trachoma clinics.

Often working alone, the nurses practiced to the limits of their nursing licenses, quickly learning how to diagnose the condition. Based on their diagnosis, they would then treat the disease according to verbal physician orders. For example, in her March 1935 report, Mary Eppich noted that she had treated four trachoma patients twice a week with "Silver Nitrate 2%" and taught them to drop "zinc solution 1% into their own eyes twice a day" on the days they did not come to clinic.[17] Covering herself legally in her report to Washington, Eppich documented: "These were the orders of Dr. Johnson when I spoke to him on March 20, 1935."[18]

In other instances, if a physician were present, the nurses worked in a more traditional role, collaborating with the visiting specialists and following their orders for treatments. For example, writing in April 1936, Gladys Solverson reported that she and Dr. Hancock had seen 93 patients in their trachoma clinic that month.[19]

TUBERCULOSIS

Tuberculosis was one of the other prevalent diseases on the Navajo reservation, and the field nurses spent much of their time identifying cases and their contacts, teaching patients and families about the disease, and driving patients to the sanatorium—if they would go or would allow a family member to go. Lillian Watson, RN, wrote of one case:

> Attempts to persuade the mother of a two-year-old boy, diagnosed with military tuberculosis, to return him to the hospital failed and it was learned that the child died in the hogan after receiving treatment by the grandfather . . . a medicine man.[20]

Negotiating the issue of hospitalization was a difficult one. The natives believed that the spirits of those who had died in a hospital remained in the hospital. They also believed that turning to a medicine man for a cure was more acceptable, in this case particularly when the medicine man was a family member. In addition to the cultural barriers, the long distances to sanatoria and the difficulties of travel provided physical hurdles to be overcome. In one of her reports, Watson described these inconveniences, noting that the nurses and physicians needed "more x-ray facilities" and "sanatoria right here on the reservation" so that families could "visit from time to time and family problems kept to a minimum."[21]

TREATING IMPETIGO

In addition to trachoma and tuberculosis, many of the Navajo suffered from impetigo, an itchy contagious skin disease characterized by blisters that gradually formed a yellow-brown crust. The infection was exacerbated by poor hygiene and inadequate diet, so treatment had to focus on the underlying causes. Mary Eppich used a combination of therapies, writing:

> Three severe cases of impetigo were found in one hogan. The treatment consists of washing with green soap, applying ammoniated mercury and bandaging. All three cases have shown much improvement. Also cod liver oil was given to them . . .[22]

MEETING BASIC NEEDS

Like so many public health nurses across the country, BIA nurse Elizabeth Forster understood that the need for food and shelter often superseded the need for medical care. On January 10, 1932, about 8 weeks after her arrival in the small trading post of Red Rock, Forster wrote to her friend that she was using food and shelter as a means of interesting the Navajo in attending the new clinic:

> Have I told you that I am having clinics once a week with a doctor out from the hospital? The weather is so cold and my people have to come from such distances that I am preparing and serving soup for them, and my dispensary, warmed by a cheerful wood fire and advertising my soup in odoriferous fashion, is a popular place on clinic day. I strongly suspect many of them come for soup and not from need to see the doctor. I am, however, by means of this bait catching a good many cases which would not otherwise come to us for care: cases of trachoma, diseased tonsils, chronic appendicitis, etc . . .[23]

PHYSICIAN REACTIONS

Whether or not the nurses saw much of the physician with whom they were assigned depended on the circumstances in which they found themselves—including not only the geographic distance from the physician, the weather, the road conditions, and the availability of physicians, but also the doctor's willingness to work with the nurses. Some, like Elizabeth Forster and Mary Eppich, worked with doctors in very cooperative arrangements. Evidence from the nurses' reports supports the fact that many doctors, working at the grass-roots level, welcomed the nurses and trusted their judgment.[24] Together the physicians and nurses visited patients in their hogans, conducted specialty clinics and surgeries, and attended meetings on the reservations. Nonetheless, one nurse had quite the opposite experience. According to Lydia King, "Our senior medical officer . . . is not in sympathy with field nurses and to quote him 'looks forward to the day when there will be no field nurses in the Navajo Area,'— it all looks pretty discouraging from where I sit."[25] Why this particular senior medical officer did not want nurses to work on the reservation is unclear, but he may have been threatened by their autonomy in practice. Later, some praised the nurses' work as they reflected on the years of collaborative practice in the Indian service. Writing to Ida Bahl, an Indian Health Service nurse in the 1970s, BIA physician Charles S. McCammon was clear about his feelings on the subject: "There has never been any question that the public health nurse . . . was and still is the backbone of Indian community health programs . . ." [26] Clearly, without nurses, many Navajo families would have been left unattended in their needs for nursing and medical care.

GAINING THE ACCEPTANCE OF THE MEDICINE MEN

One of the most difficult tasks the nurses had to undertake in the Indian health service was that of negotiating their role between the White American contract doctors and the Navajo medicine men. The field nurses, trained in traditional nursing programs throughout the United States, accepted without question the validity and efficacy of scientific American medicine.[27] Now, working on the reservation, they began to realize the importance of understanding the Navajo culture and its value of maintaining balance and order. Indeed, accepting their cultural values would be important to establishing a sense of trust. Thus, many of the BIA nurses accepted the fact that Navajo traditional healing ceremonies were at the core of their health beliefs and had to be incorporated into the treatment the nurses recommended. Delores Young, who worked as a public health nurse in Tuba City, Arizona, commented on that fact: "With the younger Indians who were undecided as to which medicine was the best, it was important to let them have both if they wanted it."[28] Another BIA nurse, Mary Zillatas, noted that she "tried to show the Indians that both cultures could be used to their advantage."[29] Both of these nurses worked according to recommendations in the *Meriam Report*: "The position taken . . . is that the work with and for the Indians must give consideration to the desires of the individual Indians."[30]

Rather than force "White man's medicine" on the Navajo, the field nurses tried to establish a sense of trust within the Navajo community so that they then could introduce Anglo-American medicine, culture, health practices, and health beliefs. The first step in this process was for the *nurse* to accept the Navajo culture. The Navajo believed that "the system of life is one inter-connected whole" and that "the whole human creature—body, mind and spirit," should be treated.[31] This holistic perspective resonated with nurses. Nonetheless, there were some significant aspects of the Navajo culture that were foreign to the increasingly scientific American nursing practice in the first half of the 20th century. A major component of the Navajo medicine men's treatment involved "Sings," or "Chantways"—ceremonial chants sung over the patient.[32] One of these, called "Beauty Way," was meant to restore balance to the patient, and was based on the Navajo belief that an imbalance in any area of a person's life could cause illness.[33] Other ceremonial Chantways included "Lifeway, Blessingway, Enemyway, the Night Chant, the Mountain Way, and Shooting Way." Different chants were meant to cure different illnesses: A Shooting Way ceremony might be used to cure an illness thought to have been caused by a snake, lightening, or an arrow; a Lifeway was used to cure an illness caused by an accident; and so on.[34]

In an attempt to show respect for the Navajo culture, some BIA nurses did not interfere with the "sings" even though they may have wanted to impose their own recommendations. Dorothy Williams recounted one visit to a hogan to see a child with a broken leg, noting:

> . . . I advised hospital for child [sic] but the family said they had already sent for the medicine man and would send the child to hospital in a few days if he failed to cure the leg. I visited the hogan a few days later and found they were still having a "Sing."[35]

While she may have been discouraged by the parents' refusal to send the child to the hospital immediately, Williams did not press the issue and instead waited for the medicine men to decide to do something different. Sometimes they did, turning to White man's medicine as a last resort. Others accepted the nurses' therapy as an adjunct treatment to their chants. As a result, the nurses often negotiated a treatment regimen somewhere between that recommended by the contract doctor and that prescribed by the Hitachi.[36] Mary Eppich described one such case: "[a baby] age 1 year, also has symptoms of Catarrhal Fever. A Sing is being held over him. My treatment was Castor Oil and Aspirin Grains 1 every four hours, plenty of water and not much food . . ."[37] Clearly, Eppich recognized the legitimate power of the medicine men within the community and the importance of working *with* them rather than undermining their authority. Other nurses did the same. Gladys Solverson described the results of that collaboration, noting:

> It has been gratifying to realize that we have gained the confidence of several of the better known medicine men. We have been called

frequently this month by the medicine men, both to their own homes as well as to "sings," to consult regarding their patients. Frequently the medicine man has advised the family to consider hospital care when we recommended it. We have brought in a good number of patients who had never seen the inside of a hospital before.[38]

The Hitachi's cooperation was essential to any consideration of hospitalization, and sometimes that cooperation was forthcoming. Many of the medicine men believed that White man's medicine was better in curing what they referred to as "White men's diseases"—whooping cough, small pox, measles, tuberculosis, and so on.[39]

Recently we advised an influential medicine man to hospitalize his 13 year old boy. The boy had been sick six days and had a temperature of 104 degrees. A "sing" was in progress and several medicine men were present. After a discussion of about an hour and a half, the medicine men decided to send the patient to the hospital . . .[40]

In her final report to the National Association of Indian Affairs in 1933, Elizabeth Forster wrote:

I believe that the Red Rock Navajos were beginning to accept me as a friend. . . . It was gratifying to have them voluntarily invite me to their ceremonies and sand paintings and to find the Medicine Men very willing to cooperate on increasingly frequent occasions.[41]

Gaining the trust of these respected community leaders was essential if the nurses were to be effective.

MATERNITY SERVICES

The public health nurses were not certified nurse midwives and were careful to work within their professional boundaries. Rather than attending childbirths, the field nurses frequently transported expectant mothers to hospitals. Mollie Reebel reported one case in which she went to extremes to get the patient to the hospital rather than deliver her at home:

. . . One of the most difficult trips I have ever made was in response to a call about two o'clock one afternoon to go out and see a lady reported as having been in labor for three days with no result. The man who came for me had started before daylight on foot and after reaching the highway had caught a ride. I inquired how far the hogan was, and was assured that it was not very far. Maybe six miles off the highway, and about twelve miles up the highway. . . . I took Laura Sherman with me for interpreter and with the Indian man as guide, we started out. After we left the highway we went sixteen miles. Again over places where there was not even a wagon road. Found the patient in terrible condition, put her in the car and headed for Ship Rock where we arrived at 7 pm having covered sixty-four miles from Nava. The patient was given immediate attention and is now recovering . . .[42]

Instead of serving as midwives, the BIA nurses worked as public health nurses, teaching the expectant and new mothers how to sew layettes for their infants, how to bathe their babies and care for their skin, how to prevent infantile diarrhea (which was prevalent on the reservation), and how to provide a more nutritious diet for their children. The nurses also conducted prenatal clinics and followed mothers and babies after the delivery, frequently treating infected and bleeding umbilical cords.[43]

THE 1940s AND 1950s

As World War II engulfed American's energy and tapped the country's resources, fewer funds were available for the Indian programs. However, the public health services continued, albeit with shortages in personnel.[44]

During the 1940s, advances in medicine brought other changes to the BIA health services. Care of infectious diseases improved as new drugs such as the sulfonamides and penicillin became available. Mobile x-ray units were instituted to screen for tuberculosis, and hospitals specializing in the treatment of tuberculosis and crippled children opened in Salt Lake City.[45]

In 1955, Congress transferred medical care from the BIA to the United States Public Health Service (USPHS). By then, the entire Indian Health Service was more structured. "By 1955, the Bureau had entered into contracts for care of Indians in 65 general community hospitals, 16 tuberculosis hospitals, and 5 mental hospitals. It also was paying for care on a fee basis at more than 180 additional general or specialized non-Indian hospitals. The policy adopted in 1952 was that the Indian Health facilities would be closed whenever 'other similar facilities are available to the eligible Indians without segregation.' . . ."[46]

By the 1950s, some of the educational efforts undertaken by the BIA nurses in the 1920s and 1930s were beginning to show positive outcomes. In a September 1957 report, one nurse (unidentified) documented that the mothers in Window Rock had become very "diarrhea-conscious"—aware of the "great killer of Navajo babies."[47] However, even with increased funding and a new bureaucratic structure, the field nurses continued to face many of the same challenges they had faced for decades. Some things did not change. As Watson reported:

> Many problems are here. We have all repeated them many times . . . about automobiles not adapted to sand dunes and mud, about our moving population, about the distances we travel, about the lack of water and sanitary facilities, about our need for more x-ray facilities, about our need for [TB] sanatoria right here on the reservation so that families can visit . . . about the need for tonsillectomies and hearing devices for children . . . and about so many other things we hardly know where to stop . . . [48]

CONCLUSION

In the first half of the 20th century, field nurses working for the BIA in the Four Corners region of the United States had to negotiate not only the extremes of weather, the great distances between patients, and the harsh environmental conditions, but also the Navajo culture in order to do effective health promotion, disease treatment, and disease prevention. Working to the full extent of their education and expertise, they often stretched the boundaries of their scope of nursing practice, particularly when they were left on their own. Navigating dust storms, blizzards, and gully washouts, as well as coping with various physician reactions to their work and learning to collaborate with the native medicine men, the nurses worked effectively to bring medical and nursing services to this underserved rural population.

NOTES

1. Elizabeth Forster to Laura Gilpin, "Correspondence" (August 1, 1932). Original correspondence published in Martha A. Sandweiss, *Denizens of the Desert: A Tale in Word and Picture of Life among the Navaho Indians* (Albuquerque, NM: University of New Mexico, 1988), 102.

2. The Navajo had been scattered throughout the Four Corners Region, where Colorado, New Mexico, Utah, and Arizona meet, accessed April 20, 2006, www.logoi. com/note/long_walk.html.

3. "Field Nurses' Narrative Reports," National Archives Records Administration, Washington, DC (hereafter cited as NARA), Bureau of Indian Affairs Record Group 75, (hereafter cited as RG75), E779, box 9 [no folders].

4. Elizabeth Forster to Emily, February 20, 1932, in Martha Sandweiss, *Denizens of the Desert,* 70.

5. Mollie Reebel, "Field Nurse's Narrative Report, April 1933," NARA, RG75, E779, box 9, [no folders].

6. Gladys Solverson, "Field Nurse's Narrative Report, March 1936," NARA, RG75, E779, box 9 [no folder]. Solverson was a nurse in the Western Navajo Area, Tuba City.

7. Dorothy Williams, RN. "Field Nurse's Narrative Reports, February and March 1936," NARA, RG75, E779, box 9. [no folders].

8. Ruth Raup, "The Indian Health Program from 1800 to 1955," Northern Arizona University, Cline Library Special Collections and Archives Department (hereafter cited as NAU-CL), Manuscript (hereafter cited as MS) 269, box 3, folder 217.

9. Lewis Meriam, *The Problem of Indian Administration* (hereafter cited as *The Meriam Report*) (Baltimore, MD: Johns Hopkins Press, 1928), 20.

10. *The Meriam Report*, 1928, 201.

11. Dorothy I. Williams, RN, "Field Nurse's Narrative Report, March 1936," NARA, RG75, E779, box 9 [no folders]. Williams worked at Teec Nos Pas in the Northern Navajo Agency. Teec Nos Pas, meaning "Trees in a Circle" in Navajo, takes its name from the cottonwoods that grow at the trading posts remote Northeast Arizona location.

12. Mary Eppich, "Field Nurse's Narrative Report, May 1935," NARA, RG75, E779, box 9, [no folders].

13. Emily K. Abel, "'We are left so much alone to work out our own problems': Nurses on American Indian Reservations during the 1930s," *Nursing History Review* 4 (1996): 43–64 (quote 49).

14. Elizabeth Forster, "Field Nurse's Narrative Report, April 1933," NARA, RG75, E779, box 9 [no folders].

15. Nena Seymour, "Field Nurse's Narrative Report, May 1935," NARA, RG 75, E779, box 9 [no folders].

16. Seymour, "Report, May 1935."

17. Eppich, "Report, March 1935." Eppich practiced in Shiprock, New Mexico, for further reading on silver nitrate, see Stella Goostray, *Drugs and Solutions for Nurses*, 2nd ed. (New York, NY: Macmillan, 1929), 55.

18. Eppich, "Report, March 1935."

19. Solverson, "Report, April 1936."

20. Lillian G. Watson, "Narrative, November 1955," Virginia Brown, Ida Bahl, and Lillian Watson Collection, 1922–1994, North Arizona University, Cline Library Special Collections and Archives Department (hereinafter cited as BBW-NAU), MS 269, pp. 1–2 (quote, p. 2).

21. Lillian Watson, "Annual Narrative Report" (March 1955–July 1956): 1–3, (quote, p. 3). NAU, Cline Library, L. Watson Collection.

22. Solverson, "Report, April 1936."

23. Elizabeth Forster to Laura Gilpin, January 10, 1932, in Martha Sandweiss, *Denizens of the Desert* (1988), 65.

24. See for example: Eppich, "Report, January 1935."

25. Lydia T. King, "Field Nurse's Narrative Report, April 30, 1936," NARA, RG75, E779, box 9 [no folders].

26. Charles S. McCammon, MD, to Ida Bahl, April1, 1974. NAU-BBWC. MS 269, box 1, folder 1.4.

27. Emily K. Abel and Nancy Reifel, chap. 26: "Interactions between Public Health Nurses and Clients on American Indian Reservations during the 1930s," in Judith Leavitt, *Women and Health in America*, 2nd ed. (Madison, WI: University of Wisconsin Press, 1999): 489–507.

28. Delores Young, Indian Health Services Nursing Questionnaire (hereafter cited as: IHSNQ), NAU-BBWC, folder 1.4.

29. Mary Zillatas, IHSNQ.

30. Meriam, *The Meriam Report* (1928), 88.

31. Lori Arviso Alvord, MD, and Elizabeth C. Van Pelt, *The Scalpel and the Silver Bear* (New York, NY: Bantam Books, 1999). See also: Mary Zillatas, IHSNQ, NAU-BBWC. MS 269, box 1, folder 1.4.

32. Mark Bahti, *A Guide to Navajo Sand Paintings* (Tucson, AZ: Rio Nuevo, 2000).

33. Lori Alvord and Elizabeth Van Pelt, *Scalpel and the Silver Bear* (1999), 186.

34. Alvord and Van Pelt, *Scalpel and the Silver Bear* (1999), 6.

35. Dorothy Williams, "Field Nurse's Narrative Report, August 1935," NARA, RG 75, E779, box 9, [no folders]. Williams practiced in the Shiprock District.

36. Charlotte J. Frisbie, *Navajo Medicine Bundles or Jish: Acquisition, Transmission and Disposition in the Past and Present* (Albuquerque, NM: University of New Mexico Press, 1987), 4–5.

37. Eppich, "Report, April 1935." See also Williams, "Report, June 1935."

38. Solverson, "Report, April 1936."

39. Robert Trennert, *White Man's Medicine: Government Doctors and the Navajo, 1863–1955* (Albuquerque, NM: University of New Mexico Press, 1998), 33.

40. Trennert, *White Man's Medicine*, 33.

41. Forster, "Report, May 1933."

42. Mollie B. Reebel, "Report, April 1933," 2.

43. Seymour, "Report, May 1935."

44. Young, IHSNQs, NAU-BBWC. MS 269, box 1.

45. Young, IHSNQs, NAU-BBWC. MS 269, box 1.

46. Raup, "The Indian Health Program," 9.

47. Monthly Narrative 1957, NAU-BBWC, MS 269, box 7, folder 437. TB remained a problem in the 1950s among the Native Americans.

48. Lillian Watson, Annual Report, BBW-NAU, MS 269, 3.

• • • • •

Conclusion

• • • • •

RURAL AMERICA HAS "... A SPECIFIC HISTORY and defining characteristics that represent a unique health care delivery environment."[1] This book set out to describe and analyze the history of nursing in rural areas of the United States during the first half of the 20th century, demonstrating how nurses shaped rural health care delivery. Using nine case studies representing select areas of the country and specific ethnic groups, the book shows how nurses brought modern health services and health education to citizens in remote rural regions of the country at a time when most rural communities had little or no public health infrastructure and little or no access to physicians.[2]

Using an historical perspective, the case studies highlight the central role that nurses played in providing access to care for rural citizens.[3] They also illustrate how nurses practiced to the full extent of their education and training and within their full scope of practice, just as the Institute of Medicine has recently recommended.[4] Rural nurses in the past, as they do today, worked as "expert generalists." Self-reliance, ingenuity, the negotiation of professional boundaries, and "doing what had to be done" were hallmarks of their practice. Challenges included those resulting from inadequate roads, extremes in weather, poor transportation, and the lack of an adequate public health infrastructure, as well as a dearth of financial, medical, and professional resources.

Working in the borderlands of race, class, and ethnic boundaries, rural nurses, company nurses, city nurses working in migrant camps, and nurse-midwives completed health assessments; immunized communities against typhoid, polio, diphtheria, and other infectious diseases; taught nutrition and sanitation; held prenatal and well-child clinics; and provided direct patient care when necessary. In rural Maine, Red Cross Town and Country nurses traveled by boat from island to island, providing health teaching and dental and medical care—doing whatever had to be done. In Virginia, school nurses served as a link between children and their families and the health department and local physicians, identifying physical defects, dental problems, and illnesses, and connecting the children and their families to care. Company nurses, providing care for workers in the cotton mill towns of Virginia, also found themselves delivering social services in addition to health care. In West Virginia, coal town nurses managed trauma, provided public health care, and served as social workers in "the company towns," thus blurring boundaries between health and social services as they struggled to deal with the social determinants of health. In West Texas, a sole physician and his nurse wife provided care to the entire oil field community, addressing emergencies and preventive care as the need arose and "making do" with what they had on hand. In Leslie County, Kentucky, nurses working in the Frontier Nursing Service provided care in patients' homes and through a decentralized system of creek-side clinics (what would be known today as primary care clinics or community health centers). Guided by standing physician orders, the nurse-midwives attended home births, managed well-baby care, and treated everything from gunshot wounds to diphtheria. On the Navajo reservation, Indian Health Service nurses practiced autonomously to treat patients with a wide range of illnesses—from colds and impetigo to pneumonia and tuberculosis. They also worked in the traditional nursing role, holding well-baby clinics and teaching principles of infant and child-care, sanitation, and nutrition. The same could be said about public health nurses working in the Farm Security Administration migratory labor camps during the Great Depression. There the nurses worked at the full extent of their scope of practice, even venturing into territory traditionally reserved for social workers as they attempted to meet the migrants' needs for food, clothing, and shelter. At the same time, they too maintained the time-honored nursing role, teaching pre- and postnatal care and promoting health as best they could.

As always, we can learn from the past, and these rural case studies, set in another time and another place, provide significant lessons. Chief among these lessons is the importance of context—the larger cultural, social, economic, and geographical setting in which nurses and physicians practice. Place matters. Culture matters. The availability of resources matters. Second among the lessons is the importance of the response to health care needs that nurses and physicians make within that context. In that regard, ingenuity, self-reliance, creative problem solving, and using the full extent of one's knowledge matter. Community participation and community acceptance also matter. An examination of the importance of each of these variables follows.

Place matters. In the current health care environment the Patient Protection and Affordable Care Act (ACA) offers the opportunity for the nation to address some of the health care disparities in rural America by providing rural citizens, many of whom live in poverty, with health insurance and/or expanded Medicaid benefits. These opportunities are not universal, however; citizens living in states whose legislators have chosen *not* to accept expanded Medicaid benefits under the ACA will not have the same opportunities as those who live in states that have. For others, limited computer access may preclude enrollment in the new ACA programs. The lack of a nearby primary care clinic or the absence of local health care providers in certain locales may also restrict equality in health care.

Citizens living in the nation's rural areas will also continue to face environmental challenges as they seek medical and nursing services. By virtue of place, geographic access to care will continue to be a challenge as rough terrain, lack of public transportation, extreme weather conditions, hazardous mountain roads, and long distances interfere. As was true in the Frontier Nursing Service, using a decentralized system of clinics may be one solution that could be recycled to facilitate access to health care in rural areas today. Critical access hospitals are also helping to solve the problem, with their focus on the stabilization of acutely ill patients and their transfer to regional medical centers, as well as the provision of lower-acuity and preventive services.[5]

Culture matters. It is essential that health care providers are culturally sensitive and able to negotiate cultural differences to arrive at an outcome that is acceptable to patients and their families. The nurses in these 20th-century case studies exemplify those values. From cooperating with the Navajo medicine men in Arizona to negotiating the cultural divide in Appalachia, coaxing resistant "old-school" European immigrants in Wisconsin, or migrant families in California to accept new ideas, early 20th-century nurses bridged cultural differences to provide care. Traditionally serving as advocates for social justice, these nurses reached a heterogeneous population in remote areas of the country to provide quality health care to all citizens—regardless of race, ethnic origin, or social class.

Ingenuity, self-reliance, creative problem solving, and using the full extent of one's knowledge also matter. It is not useful to adhere to rigid regulations or rules that simply don't make sense within the context of a given situation. In West Texas, for example, Judy Sherrod sometimes expanded her scope of practice, blurring the boundaries between medicine and nursing to provide necessary care, and—as was evidenced in the ironing board transport incident—adopted innovative solutions to "do what had to be done." The nurses working on the Navajo reservation, the migrant camp nurses in California, and the Frontier Nurses in Kentucky also did what they had to do, for the most part following standing orders, but often diagnosing and treating patients on their own.

Community participation and *community acceptance* matter. A common theme woven through all of the case studies, implicitly if not explicitly, is the importance of the nurse or other health care provider seeking input from the community about their needs, incorporating community citizens into fund raising and health promotion activities, and establishing a sense of trust with patients and their families. Coal town nurses understood this and emphasized the "culture of safety" that was important to miners and their families; mill-town nurses sought to improve working conditions and sanitation in the town; frontier nurses sought help from the locals in building the clinics; Indian health service nurses collaborated with the medicine men and showed them respect; while public health nurses in Wisconsin, Virginia, Maine, and California struggled to understand the specific needs of diverse populations.

Finally, the *availability of resources* matters. Lillian Wald was correct in advocating for the development of an "extensive and systematically organized service.. [for] the scattered dwellers in rural regions."[6] In the first half of the 20th century, the Town and Country Nursing Service (and its later iterations) worked under the direction of the American Red Cross to provide a well-organized infrastructure to support health care delivery in rural areas. Today, the American Red Cross is focused primarily on disaster preparedness and response, rather than on providing routine public health services, and the U.S. Public Health Service fills the gap. However, federal budget cuts have undermined the USPHS infrastructure and shortages in the public health nurse workforce persist. The challenge of attracting health care providers to rural areas also remains a problem.

Last but not least, as our colleagues Pat D'Antonio, Cynthia Connolly, Barb Mann Wall, Jean Whelan, and Julie Fairman argue: "History matters."[7] To paraphrase their argument, each of these case studies, examining nurses' work in different times and places and based on different primary sources, provides a rich understanding of "factors and forces" that influenced rural nursing in the past, and helps us understand the complex nature of rural nursing, past and present. Indeed, the cases bring rural nursing concepts to life and provide an historical perspective that allows for critical examination of the importance of context. In historical analysis, a century is not a very long time, and the problems of 100 years ago persist today. People all over the country—but particularly in isolated rural areas and in the "invisible" migrant camps where an undocumented workforce labors—are still seeking health care that is safe, affordable, and of high quality, just as they did in the past. To that end, Frontier Nursing Service leader Mary Breckinridge's slogan, capturing the essence of rural health care, can be recycled for use today. She noted: Our goal in providing access to health care for the nation's rural communities should be that we leave "no territory uncovered and no people uncared for."[8]

NOTES

1. Amy Elizondo and Alan Morgan, chap. 3: "The History of Rural Public Health in America," in *Rural Populations and Health: Determinants, Disparities and Solutions*, eds. Richard Crosby, Monica Wendel, Robin Vanderpool and Baretta Casey (San Francisco, CA: Jossey-Bass, 2013), 40.

2. Elizondo and Morgan, *Rural Populations and Health*, 40.

3. Arlene Keeling and Sandra Lewenson, "A Nursing Historical Perspective on the Medical Home: Impact on Health Policy," *Nursing Outlook* 61, no. 5 (July, 2013): 360–66.

4. Institute of Medicine (IOM), *The Future of Nursing: Leading Change, Advancing Health* (Washington, DC: The National Academies Press, 2010).

5. Jean Shreffler-Grant, "Acceptability: One Component in Choice of Health Care Provider," chap. 14 in *Rural Nursing: Concepts, Theory, and Practice*, ed. Charlene Winters, 4th ed. (New York, NY: Springer Publishing Company, 2013).

6. Lillian Wald to Jacob Schiff, 1910 correspondence, cited in Lavinia L. Dock, Sarah Pickett, Fannie Clement, Elizabeth Fox, and Ann Van Meter, *History of American Red Cross Nursing* (New York, NY: Macmillan, 1922), 1213.

7. Patricia D'Antonio, Cynthia Connolly, Barbra Mann Wall, Jean Whelan, and Julie Fairman, "Histories of Nursing: The Power and the Possibilities." *Nursing Outlook* (July/August, 2010): 207–13 (quote, p. 207).

8. Mary Breckinridge, *Wide Neighborhoods* (Lexington, KY: The University Press of Kentucky, 1952), 228.

Index